Few areas of medicine remain unaffected by the rapid
developments in molecular genetics that have taken place
over recent years. Not only the classic Mendelian disorders,
but also diseases of complex and multifactorial aetiology are
now susceptible to investigation at the DNA level.
Nevertheless, many clinicians remain baffled by the
technical and theoretical issues involved, and uncertain of
the implications for their field of practice. The aim of this
book is to explain, clearly and concisely, the technology and
applications of molecular genetics in those areas of clinical
medicine where they have had most impact.

Professor Brock begins his book with a basic introduction
to genetic terminology and an overview of Mendelian
principles, gene structure and gene function. He then leads
on to a description of the essential technical aspects of
molecular genetics, and the various ways in which both
normal and mutant genes can be recognized and tracked
through families and populations. The implications of the
new techniques are explored, and the potential for
diagnosis, management and treatment of a variety of human
diseases is discussed. In the final chapter, the impact of the
human genome project on modern medicine is considered.
Line diagrams and illustrations are used generously
throughout, to clarify and enliven the principles and
procedures discussed in the text.

This book will serve as a much-needed source of reference
and explanation for students and practitioners in all medical
disciplines who wish to increase their understanding of
molecular genetics in a clinical context. It will be of
particular use to clinicians in general medicine, as well as to
those in oncology, pathology, haematology, obstetrics,
paediatrics and public health.

Molecular genetics for the clinician

Molecular genetics for the clinician

D. J. H. BROCK

Professor of Human Genetics
The University of Edinburgh, U.K.

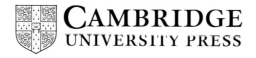

Published by the Press Syndicate of the University of Cambridge
The Pitt Building, Trumpington Street, Cambridge CB2 1RP
40 West 20th Street, New York, NY 10011-4211, USA
10 Stamford Road, Oakleigh, Victoria 3166, Australia

© Cambridge University Press 1993

First published 1993

Printed in Great Britain at the University Press, Cambridge

A catalogue record for this book is available from the British Library

Library of Congress cataloguing in publication data

Brock, D. J. H.
Molecular genetics for the clinician / D. J. H. Brock.
      p.   cm.
Includes index.
ISBN 0-521-41179-3 (hardback). – ISBN 0-521-42325-2 (pbk)
1. Medical genetics.   2. Molecular genetics.   3. Genetic
disorders.   I. Title.
[DNLM: 1. Genetics, Biochemical.   2. Hereditary Diseases –
genetics.
3. Neoplasms – genetics. QZ 50 B864m]
RB155.B66 1993
616'.042 – dc20 92-9574 CIP

ISBN 0 521 41179 3 hardback
ISBN 0 521 42325 2 paperback

CONTENTS

CONTENTS

PREFACE

Like many of my fellow human geneticists I am often asked to lecture
to medical audiences on the general theme of 'the impact of molecular
genetics on . . .', with the specialty being variously general medicine,
paediatrics or obstetrics. Recently, surgery, pathology and
haematology have been added to the list. This indicates an awareness
that something rather special is happening in molecular genetics and
that it is beginning to impinge on most if not all medical disciplines.
Quite what is happening and why it is important has eluded the bulk
of those practising clinicians who qualified before about 1980. My
lectures are often generously received; usually more generously than
they deserve, as I rush through the principles of recombinant DNA
analysis and arrive breathlessly in the last few minutes at specific
applications. Inevitably the question follows: 'What do you recom-
mend as follow-up reading?'.

The difficulty is that neither of the two types of suggested further
reading is really appropriate. The specialist books are exactly that,
loaded with detail, often superbly illustrated, but directed at the
laboratory scientist and in an unfamiliar jargon. The lay books are
either enthusiastic and superficial or weighed down by grim warn-
ings of the ethical nightmares that we are about to enter. There is very
little in between; the type of book that could be recommended to
practising doctors without blinding them with science in the first few
pages or frustrating their intellects with immature sociology as they
skim to the end.

It is, of course, an arrogance to believe that one can adequately fill
such an obvious gap, but no book is ever written by the truly humble.
What I have tried to do in the chapters that follow is to put myself in
the shoes of a doctor who qualified before 1980 (or before 1990 for
some of our more conservative medical schools) and to ask what he or
she needs to know to make sense of molecular genetics. This consists
mainly of deciding what to leave out, where to skim and where to go
for the meat of the subject. My judgements will inevitably seem

xi

perverse to some and plain wrong to others. I can only hope that somewhere there will be a readership who will find this book useful, and above all who will be stimulated to pursue the quest for deeper understanding of a subject that they will be increasingly called upon to master.

Edinburgh   D. J. H. Brock
April 1992

1 INTRODUCTION

The study of medical genetics has proceeded in a series of overlapping phases, with each phase adding new dimensions to the power of analysis. The rediscovery at the turn of the century of Mendelian principles permitted a description of the rules of simple inheritance and an understanding that some characters and diseases could be determined by single genes. These principles continue to be a dominating aspect of medical genetics, as evidenced by the name of the subject's most influential textbook, Victor McKusick's *Mendelian Inheritance in Man* (Johns Hopkins University Press, Baltimore, MD). Now in its ninth edition (1990), it is a catalogue of human traits, both normal and abnormal, that appear to follow laws of independent assortment. It is organized according to whether transmission shows autosomal dominant, autosomal recessive or X-linked inheritance, and now contains nearly 5000 entries.

The second phase of medical genetics, beginning in the late 1940s, had its origin in a belated recognition of the relationship between genes and proteins. In fact, the foundations of this subject – biochemical genetics – were laid by Sir Archibald Garrod soon after the rediscovery of Gregor Mendel's Laws of Inheritance in the early 1900s. In a series of classic papers he pointed out that the rare disorder alkaptonuria was the consequence of a discontinuity in metabolism, in all probability resulting from an inherited deficiency in a specific enzyme. The exact relationship between gene and enzyme, implicit in Garrod's writing, was not formulated until 1941. In 1949 Linus Pauling and colleagues showed that the mutant gene responsible for sickle cell anaemia produced an alteration in the structure of the haemoglobin molecule and could be demonstrated directly by gel electrophoresis. Mutant genes could therefore be studied not only through gross phenotypic change but also through their encoded protein products.

Human cytogenetics have been a comparatively late arrival on the scene. It was not until 1956 that the human diploid chromosome complement was correctly determined to be 46, and not until 1959 that the first human chromosome abnormality, trisomy 21, was described. As with biochemical genetics, the slow start of cytogenetics was technical rather than conceptual, for P. J. Waardenberg had predicted that Down syndrome would be an example of chromosomal non-disjunction in 1932. The problems of preparation and staining of human metaphase chromosomes were not really overcome until the invention by T. Caspersson of banding techniques in 1968. Within a few years it was possible to describe the normal karyotype with such precision that idiograms could be constructed showing each chromosome to be a reproducible system of regions, bands and subbands. The list of published chromosome abnormalities now exceeds that of known Mendelian conditions.

The nature of the genetic material as DNA emerged in the mid 1940s, and in 1953 James Watson and Francis Crick published their model of the physical structure of double-stranded DNA and proposed a mechanism for its replication. Another 20 years passed before technologies emerged for analysing and manipulating individual genes, the era of molecular genetics. The reason for the impasse was the considerable chemical homogeneity of different sequences of DNA, founded in different arrangements of just four nucleotide bases. But once techniques had been found for the reproducible analysis of DNA, the discovery of restriction enzymes being perhaps the most fundamental, the rate of progress in dissecting the human genome has been truly astonishing. The gene encoding placental lactogen was the first human gene to be cloned, in 1977, and within ten years it was possible to discuss realistically a project for sequencing all 3×10^9 base-pairs of the entire genome.

Molecular genetics thus represents the most recent phase in the study of genetic and quasi-genetic diseases. It is also undoubtedly the most powerful. None the less, it should not be forgotten that late-starting sciences benefit from the experience of their predecessors, and part of the reason for the rapid advances in molecular genetics comes from the existence of solid foundations and continued progress in Mendelian genetics, biochemical genetics and cytogenetics. But where DNA technology is unique and different from classic genetic technology is in its growing ability to move out of the relatively narrow constraints of single gene disorders into virtually all medical specialties. The main impact to date has been in illuminating the molecular basis of cancer (Chapter 6). Promising progress is now being made in a range of other common diseases (Chapter 8) not usually thought of as genetic. As the Human Genome Project unfolds

2

(Chapter 9), there seems little doubt that molecular genetics will become an essential science for all medical investigation.

In order to understand this new science it is necessary to have a grasp of the laboratory procedures that drive it forward. This is most easily achieved by concentrating in the first instance on single gene disorders, and by exploring the ways in which the mutational basis of Mendelian disorders can be analysed. Much of the early part of this book deals with this theme and uses the familiar examples of the haemoglobinopathies, cystic fibrosis, the muscular dystrophies and the haemophilias to illustrate methods of gene dissection and tracking. I make no apologies for this emphasis; it is an essential part of understanding what has come to be known as the new genetics. But thereafter, it is possible to begin to use the same principles and methodologies to tackle the more substantial problems of chromosome abnormalities, cancer and the common multifactorial disorders. As the twentieth century comes to an end, it is these diseases, rather than the Mendelian disorders, that will increasingly become the province of the molecular geneticist.

2 GENETIC DISEASES

The term genetic disease is broad and includes disorders in which aberrations in the genetic material are entirely responsible for the pathology as well as those in which genetic factors are only partly and obscurely involved. Conventionally, the spectrum of genetic diseases is divided into three major categories:

1 *Mendelian disorders* (also referred to as single-gene defects, monogenic disorders or single-locus disorders) are caused by a mutant allele or pair of mutant alleles at a single genetic locus. They may be inherited or be the result of new mutations. When inherited, the transmission patterns are simple and classified as autosomal dominant, autosomal recessive, X-linked dominant or X-linked recessive.

2 *Chromosome disorders* are caused by the loss, gain or abnormal arrangement of one or more of the 46 chromosomes of the diploid cell. A majority of chromosome disorders are de novo events, arising from major mutations in the parents' germ cells. There are also examples of inherited chromosomal aberrations, showing modified patterns of Mendelian transmission.

3 *Multifactorial disorders* include many of the common diseases of adulthood as well as a majority of congenital malformations. They are thought to involve interactions between genes and environmental factors, although the number and nature of both genes and environmental factors are poorly understood. Occurrence and recurrence risks are estimated empirically.

To these three major categories of genetic disease, advances in molecular biology have now added another two:

4 *Somatic genetic disorders* are mutations in the genetic material that arise in specific somatic cells, and often give rise to

4

tumours. The somatic event is not inherited, even though it involves gene mutation. However, in many cancers there is an inherited predisposition to tumour formation, and the interaction between inherited and somatic mutations can be complex. This is discussed in Chapter 6.

5 *Mitochondrial disorders* arise from mutations in the mitochondrial genome, which is quite distinct from the bulk of DNA carried by chromosomes in the cell nucleus. Mitochondrial DNA is transmitted through only the maternal line, and patterns of inheritance are different from those seen in Mendelian disorders.

Any classification of genetic diseases inevitably involves some degree of oversimplification. Some disorders, such as cleft lip and palate, anencephaly or spina bifida, usually regarded as having a multifactorial aetiology, may occasionally be inherited in an apparently Mendelian manner. Small chromosomal deletions involving several genes at adjacent loci – contiguous-gene syndromes – bridge the gap between chromosome and Mendelian disorders. Many of these examples will be discussed in later chapters. None the less, despite these exceptions and complications, the five categories listed in Table 2.1 are a useful general classification.

GENETIC TERMINOLOGY

The basic rules of simple inheritance were formulated by Gregor Mendel in 1865. Although understanding of the concepts has evolved and some of the definitions have changed, appreciation of the facts of Mendelian inheritance is important in all types of genetic disease. It is also a useful introduction to the basic terminology of genetics.

In modern form the essential features of Mendelian inheritance are:

1 Inherited characteristics or traits are determined by genes. With the exception of genes carried on the X and Y chromosomes in males, genes come in pairs, one derived from each parent. The particular form of a gene is referred to as an allele. The physical position of a gene on a chromosome is the locus. It must be noted that since most cells are diploid (have pairs of chromosomes) the term locus usually refers to a site on two homologous chromosomes (Fig. 2.1) but can also refer to the position on the single X and Y chromosomes in males.

2 When there are two identical alleles at a locus, a person is homozygous; when the alleles are different the person is

Table 2.1. *Major categories of genetic disease*

Category	Comments
Mendelian disorders	New mutations or inherited. When inherited, obey simple rules of transmission
Chromosome disorders	Usually de novo events. When inherited, often show modified pattern of Mendelian transmission
Multifactorial disorders	Exact genetic influence poorly understood. Risks estimated empirically
Somatic cell disorders	Involve mutations in somatic cells. Somatic event is not inherited
Mitochondrial disorders	Mutations in the mitochondrial genome. Transmitted through the maternal line

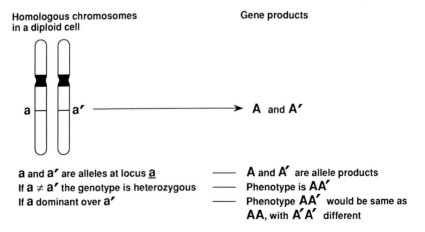

Fig. 2.1. Illustration of some important parts of genetic terminology.

heterozygous. When there is only a single copy of a gene (X and Y in males, or through part or whole chromosome loss), the situation is referred to as hemizygous.

3 The genetic constitution is the genotype. The physical expression of the genotype, whether as a grossly observable characteristic or as a specific protein, is the phenotype.

4 When one member of a pair of dissimilar alleles determines the phenotype it is referred to as a dominantly inherited characteristic. Conversely, in a recessively inherited characteristic both alleles influence the phenotype. In general, the terms dominant and recessive should be restricted to characteristics and not used to describe genes.

5 During gametogenesis, pairs of alleles separate (or segregate) into different germ cells, so that sperm and egg have a single allele at each locus, and are thus termed haploid. This was described in Mendel's *Law of Segregation*.

6 During gametogenesis, most pairs of genes (i.e. most genetic loci) behave as though they are independent of one another. This was Mendel's *Law of Independent Assortment*. We now know that genes that are close together on a chromosome do not assort independently, and this exception has been crucial to the development of human genetics.

7 Because females have two X chromosomes and males have only one, the inheritance of characteristics that are X linked is different from that of chromosomes determined by the other 22 chromosomal pairs. The same applies to the few genes carried on the Y chromosome.

PATTERNS OF MENDELIAN INHERITANCE

Disorders carried by mutant genes at a single genetic locus show one of three simple Mendelian patterns of inheritance: autosomal dominant, autosomal recessive or X-linked (which may be dominant or recessive). Since human families are often small, it may be difficult to distinguish the mode of inheritance and clinical geneticists rely heavily on McKusick's *Mendelian Inheritance in Man*. However, even in this essential reference book, genetic heterogeneity may result in a named disorder being listed under more than one heading, and the inheritance pattern in the family at risk will have to be worked out from the available clues and from the first principles of Mendelian transmission.

AUTOSOMAL DOMINANT INHERITANCE

Disorders inherited as autosomal dominants manifest in the hetero-zygous state. The affected individual carries a mutant allele on one chromosome and a normal allele on the homologous chromosome. Since the relevant locus is on one of the 22 autosomes, both males and females can be affected. Because alleles at a particular genetic locus segregate at meiosis, there is a 50% chance that the child of an affec-ted parent will be affected (Fig. 2.2).

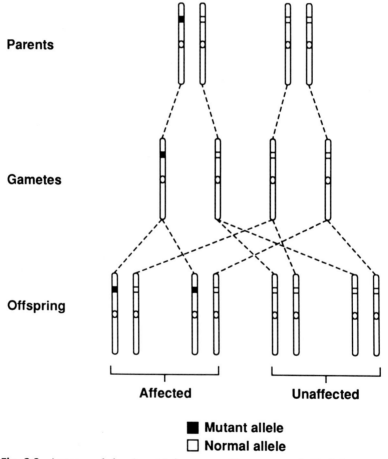

Fig. 2.2. Autosomal dominant inheritance. On average, half of the offspring of an affected parent will also be affected. Both males and females can be affected.

There are several complicating factors in autosomal dominant inheritance. The clinical expression of the disorder may be quite variable; this is referred to as expressivity, and can be a confounding factor in the description of a disease. For example, in polydactyly an affected person may have a complete extra finger or simply a modified appendage on the side of the hand. In the extreme, there may be no expression of any symptoms of the disease in a person who, from pedigree analysis, must be carrying the gene; this is referred to as non-penetrance. The degree of penetrance of a particular mutant gene can be calculated from inspection of families in which the disorder is segregating and recorded as a percentage. In contrast, expressivity is a purely descriptive term.

In many autosomal dominant conditions the severity of the disorder affects the biological fitness. In these cases the frequency of the disorder will be maintained by new mutations, occurring in the gametes of the affected person's parents. There is an inverse relationship between biological fitness and the proportion of new mutations comprising an autosomal dominant disorder. Thus in myositis ossificans, where the biological fitness is about 0.01, the proportion of new mutations may be as high as 99%. In Huntington's disease, where biological fitness is at least 0.8, very few genuine new mutations have been described.

In an autosomal dominant, the affected individual displays symptoms even with only a single dose of the mutant allele. Occasionally, since such disorders are generally rare, a person may inherit a second mutant allele at the same locus, and thus be a homozygous affected. In a true dominant, the clinical expression of the disorder will be the same in the homozygous and heterozygous affected individuals. Huntington's disease is one of the few known examples of true dominance. In other autosomal dominants, such as familial hypercholesterolaemia, homozygous affecteds have a much more severe range of symptoms than do heterozygous affecteds. This phenomenon is sometimes referred to as haploid insufficiency.

AUTOSOMAL RECESSIVE INHERITANCE

Autosomal recessive disorders are clinically apparent in only the homozygote, who has a mutant allele on each of the homologous chromosomes. Both sexes can be affected. Heterozygous carriers of a single mutant allele are clinically normal. Most affected cases arise from a mating between two heterozygotes. In such crosses there is a 25% chance of normal outcome, a 50% chance of heterozygous outcome and a 25% chance of affected outcome (Fig. 2.3).

Most autosomal recessive conditions are quite rare and may occur as isolated events in apparently normal families. The frequency of heterozygotes is always much greater. The relationship between heterozygote frequencies and the frequency of the disorder in outbred populations can be derived from the Hardy–Weinberg equilibrium. This states that if the frequency of the normal allele is p and the frequency of the mutant allele is q:

the relative proportion of normal homozygotes is p^2,
the relative proportion of affected homozygotes is q^2,
the relative proportion of heterozygotes is $2pq$.

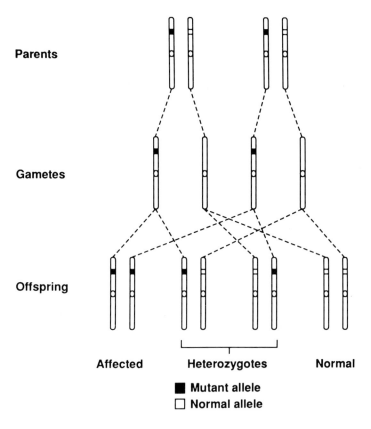

Fig. 2.3. Autosomal recessive inheritance. When each parent is a heterozygote, 25% of the offspring will be homozygous affecteds, 50% will be heterozygotes and 25% will be homozygous normals.

Table 2.2. *Heterozygote frequencies in autosomal recessive conditions*

Incidence of disorder (q^2)	Gene frequency[a] (q)	Heterozygote frequency[a] ($\sim 2q$)
1 in 1000	0.0316	0.0632
1 in 2000	0.0224	0.0447
1 in 3000	0.0183	0.0365
1 in 5000	0.0141	0.0283
1 in 10 000	0.0100	0.0200
1 in 50 000	0.0045	0.0089
1 in 100 000	0.0032	0.0064

Note: [a]These frequencies should be multiplied by 100 to give commonly quoted percentage values, e.g. 0.0316 = 3.16%.

The Hardy–Weinberg law is often used by first estimating the incidence of affected homozygotes (q^2) and then solving the other proportions by using the relationship $p=1-q$.

For example, the incidence of cystic fibrosis in the U.K. is about 1 in 2500.

Thus,

$$q^2 = 1/2500 \text{ or } 0.0004,$$
$$q = 1/50 \text{ or } 0.02,$$
$$p = 1-q = 0.98,$$

and

$$2pq = 2 \times 0.98 \times 0.02$$
$$= 0.0392 \text{ (approximately 1 in 25).}$$

Examples of heterozygote frequencies for some recessively inherited disorders are shown in Table 2.2. It is usually sufficiently accurate to assume that $p \approx 1$, and thus to estimate the heterozygote frequency as twice the frequency of the mutant allele. Only when the incidence of a genetic disorder falls below 1 in 40 000 does the heterozygote frequency drop below 1%.

The Hardy–Weinberg law applies to outbred populations where mating is assumed to be random. In communities where there is inbreeding, partners are more likely to carry identical rare recessive genes than are partners in an outbred population, and are therefore more likely to have affected children. One of the important clues to establishing a rare condition as being due to autosomal recessive inheritance is the finding of a degree of relationship (perhaps first cousins) in the parents of an affected child.

Virtually all Mendelian disorders are characterized by genetic heterogeneity: the existence of several different disease-causing mutant alleles at a particular locus. In an autosomal recessive condition, an affected individual may inherit a different allele from each parent. Although such people are regarded as homozygous affecteds because they have the disease, the correct term is compound heterozygote, since only a single dose of each different mutant allele is present at the locus in question (Fig. 2.4). The phrase compound heterozygote is often confused with double heterozygote: the latter refers to heterozygosity at distinct and different loci and in autosomal recessive conditions would not be associated with clinical disease.

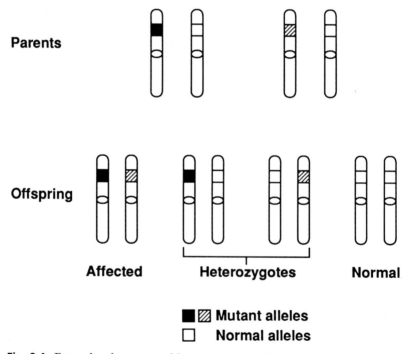

Fig. 2.4. Example of compound heterozygosity. If each heterozygous parent carries a different mutant allele at the same genetic locus, the affected individual will have two different mutant alleles and is therefore a compound heterozygote.

X-LINKED INHERITANCE

X-linked inheritance is similar to autosomal inheritance, with the critical difference that females have two X chromosomes whereas males have one. X-linked inheritance is usually recessive, the most frequent pattern being one in which a carrier mother gives birth to an affected male child. As shown in Fig. 2.5a, a mating between a normal father and a carrier mother has four possible outcomes each with 25% chance: an affected son or normal son, a carrier daughter or a normal daughter. In this pattern, the father contributes only normal X chromosomes to his daughters and Y chromosomes to his sons, and thus the carrier status of the mother is all important. However, if the father is affected, all his daughters will be carriers and all his sons will be normal (Fig. 2.5b). An affected male is termed hemizygous because he has a single X chromosome.

In order to explain the fact that females do not produce twice as much product of X-linked genes as do males, Mary Lyon proposed that in female cells only a single X chromosome was active. This phenomenon, known as X inactivation or lyonization, occurs during early embryonic life and is random, so that either paternal or maternal X chromosomes can be inactivated. Once the original X inactivation process has occurred, all the descendent cells in a particular tissue have the same X-chromosome in the inactive state (Fig. 2.6). In some mysterious fashion, the relevant chromosome is imprinted with the information that it is to stay inactivated and thus not to express any product (see Chapter 7). There are some exceptions to lyonization: several genes at the tip of the short arm of the X chromosome (in the region where pairing with the Y chromosome takes place) escape inactivation and are expressed in normal fashion.

There are several important consequences of lyonization. Rarely, female carriers of X-linked recessive disorders may show some clinical signs of the disease. An example is Duchenne muscular dystrophy. It is presumed that in such affected females the original X inactivation of progenitor muscle cells has, by chance, largely affected the normal X chromosome, and that most of the descendent muscle cells are now expressing the X chromosome carrying the mutant gene. These individuals are known as manifesting heterozygotes. Conversely, if lyonization has, in most cells, affected the X chromosome carrying the mutant allele, it will be difficult to detect the carrier state by biochemical tests, since the levels of product will be essentially normal.

Lyonization also blurs the distinction between X-linked dominant

13

(a)

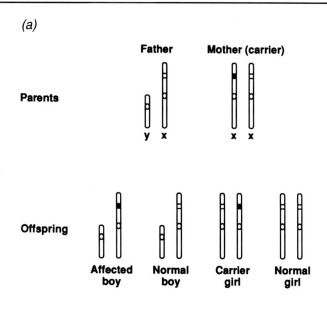

(b)

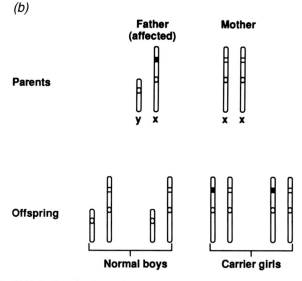

Fig. 2.5. X-linked recessive inheritance. In (*a*) the mother carries the mutant allele on one of her X chromosomes, while in (*b*) the father (who is affected) carries the mutant allele on his single X chromosome.

14

and X-linked recessive inheritance. In both cases, males, with their single X chromosome, will be affected. However, female carriers of an X-linked dominant trait may have only mild or subclinical disease if by chance their abnormal X chromosome has been preferentially inactivated. There is also a chance that cells containing the abnormal X chromosome will be selected against during proliferation of the cell line from the original precursor cell. An example of this is found in the severe X-linked recessive Lesch–Nyhan syndrome. Female carriers of this disorder all have normal levels of the gene product hypoxanthine guanine phosphoribosyl-transferase in red blood cells, presumably because cells with an abnormal X chromosome and lacking this enzyme do not survive.

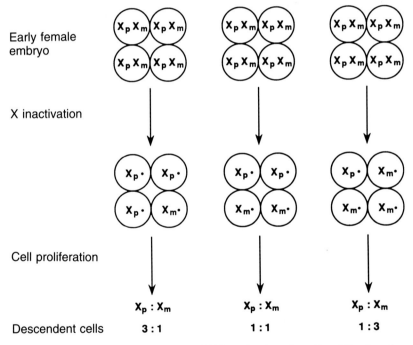

Fig. 2.6. Schematic representation of X inactivation. In cells of the female early embryo both X chromosomes (Xp and Xm) are active. X inactivation in the embryo is random, so that in different blocks of cells, variable proportions of cells contain active Xp or Xm chromosomes. The descendent lines derived from the original inactivation events retain the same proportions of active and inactive X chromosomes.

15

CODOMINANT INHERITANCE

The inheritance of virtually all Mendelian disorders can be classified as autosomal dominant, autosomal recessive or X linked. Very few diseases have been described where inheritance is Y-chromosome linked. However, even the most casual inspection of the genetics of the ABO blood group system suggests that dominance and recessiveness do not adequately describe the inheritance of blood types. Both type A and type B are dominant with respect to type O, but inheritance of type A and type B gives an intermediate AB phenotype.

This example illustrates a general truism that, when inspection of the phenotype is at the biochemical or molecular level, the terms dominant and recessive become redundant and should be replaced by codominant. This means that the product of each allele at a locus can be individually distinguished. An example of this has already been shown for compound heterozygotes in recessively inherited diseases (Fig. 2.4). There is no doubt that the disease itself is inherited as an autosomal recessive but, since the allelic products are distinguishable, they are inherited as codominants, It is therefore important to avoid talking about dominant genes (although we all do), and to recognize that it is only gross phenotypes that show dominance or recessiveness.

FREQUENCY OF MENDELIAN DISORDERS

Many Mendelian disorders are found at variable incidences in different ethnic groups, and statements on frequency must be qualified by description of the population surveyed. Sickle cell anaemia occurs at highest frequency in populations with a mid-African background, β-thalassaemia in Asiatics, and cystic fibrosis in north Europeans and their descendants. The X-linked disorder glucose-6-phosphate dehydrogenase deficiency is found at high levels in African, Asiatic and Oriental populations and in Europeans and Arabs from the Mediterranean basin. In most of the more prevalent disorders, a selective advantage favouring heterozygotes is probably responsible for high gene frequencies. In less prevalent disorders, with pockets in particular ethnic groups, a founder effect is a more likely explanation.

The frequency of the more common Mendelian disorders in the U.K. population is shown in Table 2.3. The list is restricted to diseases caused by mutant alleles at a single genetic locus and thus excludes comparatively common Mendelian forms of blindness, deafness and mental retardation, which are probably very heterogeneous. Birth

Table 2.3. *Approximate frequency of most common Mendelian disorders in the U.K. population*

Disorder	Frequency per 1000 births
Autosomal dominant	
Familial combined hyperlipidaemia	5.0
Familial hypercholesterolaemia	2.0
Dominant otosclerosis	1.0
Adult polycystic kidney disease	0.8
Multiple exostoses	0.5
Huntington's disease	0.5
Neurofibromatosis	0.4
Myotonic dystrophy	0.2
Congenital spherocytosis	0.2
Polyposis coli	0.1
Autosomal recessive	
Cystic fibrosis	0.4
α_1-Antitrypsin deficiency	0.2
Phenylketonuria	0.1
Congenital adrenal hyperplasia	0.1
Spinal muscular atrophy	0.1
Sickle cell anaemia	0.1
β-Thalassaemia	0.05
X-linked recessive	
Fragile X syndrome	0.5
Duchenne muscular dystrophy	0.3
X-linked ichthyosis	0.2
Haemophilia A	0.1
Becker muscular dystrophy	0.05
Haemophilia B	0.03

frequencies of late-onset dominantly inherited conditions are difficult to calculate from population prevalence data, and are therefore fairly rough estimates. Familial combined hyperlipidaemia, at about 1 in 200 births, is probably the most common Mendelian disorder in humans, although it is not yet clear whether it is a homogeneous entity. Cystic fibrosis is the most frequent serious autosomal recessive

Table 2.4. *Main categories of chromosome disorder*

Numerical abnormalities
  Polyploidy
  Aneuploidy
    Autosomal
    Sex chromosomes

Structural abnormalities
  Deletions
  Duplications
  Inversions
  Ring chromosomes
  Isochromosomes
  Translocations
    Reciprocal
    Robertsonian
    Insertional

condition in the U.K., though some would argue that the comparatively benign haemochromatosis (about 3 per 1000 births) should head the list. The fragile X syndrome is an example of a chromosome disorder that shows modified X-linked recessive transmission (Chapter 7).

CHROMOSOME DISORDERS
A detailed description of chromosome disorders is outside the scope of this book. None the less, the new analytical techniques of molecular genetics have begun to make a substantial impact on this group of disorders and on the biological events that precipitate cytogenetic abnormality (Chapter 7). A brief description of the major categories of chromosome disorder is therefore necessary.

There are two broad groups of chromosome abnormality, the numerical and the structural (Table 2.4). The chromosome number of the human haploid cell, i.e. mature germ cells, is 23, and of the normal diploid cell 46. A chromosome number that is an exact multiple of 23 but exceeds the normal diploid number of 46 is called polyploidy. Triploidy (69 chromosomes) is seen quite often in spontaneous abortions (or in early prenatal diagnosis), but is essentially incompatible with life. Tetraploidy (92 chromosomes) is also seen occasionally in spontaneous abortions but virtually never in liveborns.

The more common types of numerical chromosome abnormality result from the gain or loss of one or more chromosomes, and are referred to as aneuploidy. Aneuploidy is the result of non-disjunction, the failure of paired chromosomes to separate during cell division. It can occur in either the first or second divisions of meiosis (Fig. 2.7) and leads to cells with an extra copy of a chromosome (trisomy) or cells with a missing copy of a chromosome (monosomy). Aneuploidy also occurs during mitotic division and leads to a mosaic, a person whose tissues consist of a mixture of two cell lines, each line having a different chromosome complement.

The most common autosomal trisomy is that of chromosome 21, responsible for about 95% of cases of Down syndrome. Less frequent autosomal trisomies are those of chromosomes 13 and 18. Numerical abnormalities of the sex chromosomes are, in general, of less severe clinical consequence. They include 47,XYY, 47,XXY (Klinefelter syndrome), 45,X (Turner syndrome) and 47,XXX.

Structural chromosome abnormalities all result from chromosomal

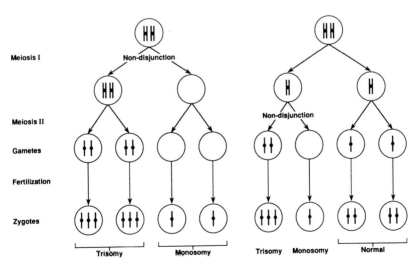

Fig. 2.7. Consequences of chromosomal non-disjunction in either the first (left side of diagram) or second (right side of diagram) meiotic divisions. A single pair of homologous chromosomes is shown. It is assumed that fertilization is by a normal gamete.

19

breakage. If only a single chromosome is involved the result may be a deletion (loss of material), duplication (gain of material) or inversion (rearrangement of material). Deletions of both ends of a chromosome followed by fusion of the 'sticky' ends can result in a ring chromosome. A simultaneous duplication and deletion leads to an isochromosome.

When chromosomal breakage involves more than one chromosome, a common result is a translocation. In reciprocal translocations, material distal to the breakage points is exchanged, either between homologous or non-homologous chromosomes (Fig. 2.8). In Robertsonian translocations, breakage near the centromere in two non-homologous acrocentric chromosomes results in a centric fusion of the long arms at a common centromere and loss from the cell of the fused short arms. In insertional translocations, material from one chromosome may be inserted into a gap in another chromosome. In all these rearrangements there is often no net loss of genetic material and the person may be a perfectly normal, balanced-translocation carrier. However, his or her offspring are at increased risk of inheriting unbalanced chromosome-constitutions.

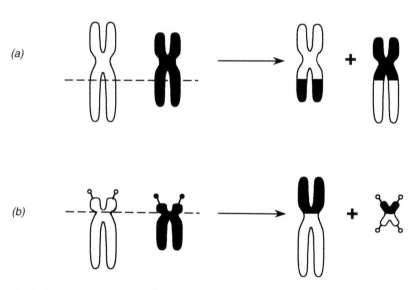

(a)

(b)

Fig. 2.8. Examples of chromosomal translocation. In a reciprocal translocation (*a*) all the material is retained in the balanced carrier. In a Robertsonian translocation (*b*) the small centric fragment is usually lost, but is normally composed of genetically inert heterochromatin.

Table 2.5. *Chromosome abnormalities in surveys of the newborn*

Abnormality	Rate per 1000 births
Sex chromosome	
47,XYY	0.47
47,XXY	0.47
45,X	0.05
47,XXX	0.52
Other	0.56
Autosomal trisomies	
Trisomy 13	0.05
Trisomy 18	0.12
Trisomy 21	1.25
Other	0.02
Balanced structural arrangements	
D/D centric fusions	0.70
D/G centric fusions	0.19
Other	1.04
Unbalanced structural arrangements	0.60
Total	6.04

Chromosomal abnormalities are very common. Some 15% to 20% of recognized pregnancies end in miscarriage and about half of the abortuses have been shown to have a major chromosome aberration. Studies on preimplantation embryos suggest that as many as 20% may have an abnormal karyotype. However, natural wastage will account for a large majority of these, and the live-birth frequency is only 0.6%. A breakdown of common chromosome abnormalities in newborn infants is shown in Table 2.5. The most serious of these is undoubtedly trisomy 21, which occurs in about 1 in about 800 births.

Although chromosome abnormalities are relatively common, most are not inherited. There is an increased incidence of the autosomal trisomies 13, 18 and 21 and of the sex-chromosome aneuploidies 47,XXX and 47,XXY with advancing maternal age, and this is most striking for trisomy 21. Affected individuals rarely reproduce, because of the gravity of the condition (trisomies 13, 18 and 21) or because of infertility (47,XXY or 45,X). Fertile individuals with sex-chromosome abnormalities (47,XXX and 47,XYY) do not appear to transmit their abnormality, for reasons that are not clear.

The exception to the general rule of non-inheritance of chromosome abnormalities is found in the clinically normal carrier of a balanced translocation. There is a theoretical risk of one in three that live offspring will have an unbalanced chromosome constitution, with part of a chromosome triplicated. However, the actual risk depends on the nature of the translocation and whether it is the father or the mother who is the balanced carrier. The risks are determined empirically and are substantially less than the theoretical value.

MULTIFACTORIAL DISORDERS

In most common adult diseases, as well as in congenital malformations, there is no suggestion of a Mendelian mode of inheritance. None the less, there are often indications that genetic factors are involved and that a complex interaction of genes and environment causes the disorder. Three lines of evidence are usually cited for including such disorders under the broad umbrella of genetic or quasi-genetic diseases.

1 The disorder may occur at higher frequencies in certain racial or ethnic groups. Since this can result from different environments, it is also necessary to show that the higher frequency persists, perhaps in a modulated form, when the group moves to a different environment.

2 The disorder may occur at a higher frequency in the immediate relatives of an affected person when compared to the frequency in the general population. First-degree relatives, i.e. siblings, children or parents, of an index case have half of their genes in common. Second-degree relatives, i.e. grandparents, grandchildren, nephews, nieces, aunts and uncles, of an index case have one-quarter of their genes in common. If a disorder shows a much higher incidence in first-degree relatives and a higher incidence in second-degree (and perhaps even third-degree) relatives compared to the incidence in the general population, this could be taken as presumptive evidence of the importance of genetic factors.

3 The best evidence comes from inspection of concordance rates in monozygotic (MZ) and dizygotic (DZ) twins. MZ

22

Table 2.6. *Twin concordance for congenital malformations and diseases of adulthood*

Disorder	Concordance (%)	
	MZ twins	DZ twins
Congenital malformations		
Cleft lip ± palate	35	5
Club foot	30	2
Congenital dislocation of hip	40	3
Pyloric stenosis	20	2
Spina bifida	6	3
Adult diseases		
Diabetes (insulin-dependent)	50	10
Hypertension	30	10
Manic depression	80	10
Multiple sclerosis	20	5
Schizophrenia	40	10
Alzheimer's disease	40	10

twins are genetically identical, whereas DZ twins have half of their genes in common. If a disorder has no genetic component, the concordance rates in MZ and DZ twins will be the same and reflect the significance of a particular environment. The greater the difference between concordance rates in MZ and DZ twins, the more probable it is that genetic factors are important. Some comparisons are shown in Table 2.6.

It must be made clear that the three lines of evidence cited above are at best indicative of a genetic predisposition to a disorder and give no clues as to the nature or number of the genes involved. Thus, the practical value of such analyses may be questioned. However, the techniques of molecular genetics now make it possible to begin systematic searches for predisposing genetic loci in such disorders (Chapter 8). Obviously it makes sense to focus such investigations on those disorders or congenital malformations in which the genetic contribution is major rather than minor. Comparison of insulin-dependent diabetes mellitus and spina bifida, for example, suggest

23

Table 2.7. *A comparison of the relative importance of genetic factors in two different multifactorial disorders*

Evidence for genetic factors	Insulin-dependent diabetes mellitus	Spina bifida
Higher frequency in certain racial and ethnic groups	Yes	Yes
Higher frequency in first and second-degree relatives	Yes	Yes
Concordance in MZ vs DZ twins	50% vs 10%	6% vs 3%

that predisposing genes are more likely to be found in the former than in the latter (Table 2.7). The main evidence for this comes from the different concordance rates in MZ and DZ twins: for spina bifida the rates are barely above the level of experimental error.

MITOCHONDRIAL INHERITANCE

Most human genes are carried on chromosomes in the nucleus of the cell and obey the Mendelian Laws of the Assortment (and usually) Independent Segregation. The exceptions are the genes of the mitochondria, which are small cytoplasmic organelles that may have originated from capture of bacteria early in evolution. Each mitochondrion has several copies of a circular chromosome composed of a comparatively small amount of DNA. Mitochondrial DNA controls a number of protein components of the respiratory chain and oxidative phosphorylation system, as well as some special types of RNA.

Mitochondrial inheritance is exclusively matrilineal, since the sperm contributes no cytoplasm to the zygote. However, whereas each nuclear chromosome is present in only two copies per cell, the mitochondrial chromosome is present in thousands of copies. In cells that have a mixture of mutant and normal mitochondrial DNA, the genotype may shift during cell replication either in the direction of the mutant or in the direction of the normal. There is some evidence that rapidly dividing cells may select against mitochondrial DNA containing deletions or major mutations. Mitochondrial DNA has a high rate of mutation and there is considerable gene variation in the normal population.

The study of mitochondrial disease is still in its infancy. A pattern of matrilineal transmission of a disorder is suggestive of mitochondrial inheritance, but is not conclusive. The strongest evidence for a mitochondrial DNA mutation in a genetic disease is in Leber's optic atrophy, characterized by late-onset bilateral loss of central vision and by cardiac dysrhythmias. No case of paternal transmission of this disorder has been documented. A point mutation in the mitochondrial gene coding for a subunit in a NADH dehydrogenase has been suggested as the primary cause, but this is yet to be confirmed. Three other disorders that may be due to mitochondrial-gene defects are myoclonus epilepsy with ragged red fibres (MERRF), mitochondrial myopathy with encephalopathy, lacticacidosis and stroke (MELAS) and Kearns–Sayre syndrome.

SUGGESTED READING

Borgaonkar, D. S. (1989). *Chromosomal Variation in Man.* 5th Edition, Alan R. Liss, New York.

Connor, J. M. and Ferguson-Smith, M. A. (1988). *Essential Medical Genetics.* 2nd Edition, Blackwell Scientific, Oxford.

Fraser-Roberts, J. A. and Pembrey, M. E. (1985). *An Introduction to Medical Genetics.* 8th Edition, Oxford University Press, Oxford.

Gardner, R. J. M. and Sutherland, G. R. (1989). *Chromosome Abnormalities and Genetic Counselling.* Oxford University Press, Oxford.

Gelehrter, T. D. and Collins, F. S. (1990). *Principles of Medical Genetics.* Williams and Wilkins, Baltimore, MD.

Harper, P. S. (1988). *Practical Genetic Counselling.* Wright, London.

McKusick, V. A. (1990). *Mendelian Inheritance in Man.* 9th Edition, Johns Hopkins University Press, Baltimore, MD.

Scriver, C. R., Beaudet, A. L., Sly, W. S. and Valle, D. (Editors) (1988). *The Metabolic Basis of Inherited Disease.* 6th Edition, McGraw–Hill, New York.

Vogel, F. and Motulsky, A. G. (1987). *Human Genetics.* 2nd Edition, Springer Verlag, Berlin.

Weatherall, D. J. (1991). *The New Genetics and Clinical Practice.* 3rd Edition, Oxford University Press, Oxford.

3 THE TECHNOLOGY OF MOLECULAR GENETICS

All genetic variation depends ultimately on mutation: physical and chemical alterations in the hereditary material. Although mutations occur in DNA, their phenotypic effects in the cell are usually caused by altered or absent RNA or proteins. Therefore a description of the role of genes in genetic diseases must examine not only the nature and structure of genes themselves, but also the way in which the information in DNA is passed on to the cell. This involves two processes: the transcription of DNA into RNA and the translation of RNA into proteins containing specific sequences of amino acid residues. The central dogma of molecular biology states that the flow of genetic information is unidirectional and that the amino acid sequence of any protein is a direct consequence of the DNA sequence in the gene that controls it. There may be some exceptions to central dogma: occasionally the coding sequence in an RNA molecule differs from the sequence of the DNA from which it is transcribed (RNA editing), but it is still a very useful general principle.

THE STRUCTURE AND FUNCTION OF GENES

By the end of the nineteenth century it was apparent that chromosomes were the carriers of the units of inheritance. The exact nature of the hereditary material emerged slowly, and for many years it seemed that proteins were more likely candidates than DNA. Experiments with transforming factors in bacteria, carried out in the 1940s, demonstrated unequivocally that DNA was the genetic material. It is now accepted that, with the exception of some viruses that use RNA as their genetic material, in virtually all species genes are made of DNA.

The acceptance of DNA as the genetic material was accelerated by the physical model for genetic transmission provided by James Watson and Francis Crick in 1953. From X-ray crystallographic data, they deduced a double-helical structure for DNA with two intertwined chains running in opposite directions (Fig. 3.1). Each DNA strand is

26

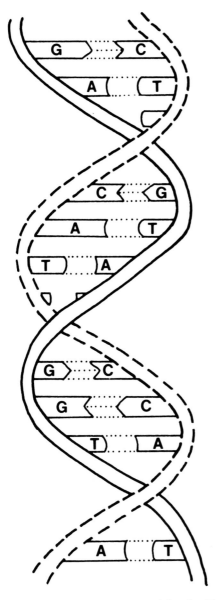

Fig. 3.1. Schematic representation of the double-helical structure of DNA. The deoxyribose–phosphate backbones are shown as ribbons and run in opposite directions. In the Watson–Crick structure, base-pairing is always between A (purine) and T (pyrimidine) or between G (purine) and C (pyrimidine).

27

composed of varying patterns of four distinct units, the nitrogenous bases, adenine, guanine, cytosine and thymine, strung in seemingly random sequence along a deoxyribose–phosphate backbone. Adenine and guanine are purine bases and cytosine and thymine are pyrimidine bases; they are usually referred to as A, G, C and T. A base linked to a sugar is called a nucleoside; when a phosphate group is added it is called a nucleotide (Table 3.1). In the Watson–Crick model, the forces holding the two DNA strands together are specific hydrogen bonds between pairs of bases, A (a purine) always bonding with T (a pyrimidine) and G (a purine) always bonding with C (a pyrimidine). Thus each strand is complementary to the other, with a sequence of AATCGG on one strand, for example, being matched by TTAGCC on the other strand. The direction of the strands is indicated as either 5' to 3' or 3' to 5', this being determined by the numbering of the carbon atoms in the deoxyribose–phosphate backbone. Apart from the absolute requirement for base-pairing between complementary strands, there are few other restrictions on the base sequence in a DNA molecule.

As pointed out by Watson and Crick, the double-helical structure of DNA, with complementary bases in opposite strands, suggests a model for the replication of the genetic material. Unwinding of the helix provides two templates for synthesis of complementary strands (Fig. 3.2). Each daughter double-stranded molecule contains one parental strand and one newly synthesized strand, a form of replication known as semi-conservative. The fidelity of sequence in the daughter strands is maintained by the all-important base-pairing requirement.

The sequence of bases in a DNA molecule represents the information content of the gene, and is critical in determining what it does. If the DNA strand is N bases in length there are 4^N possible different sequences. Human haploid cells (sperms and eggs) contain sequences of DNA of about 3.5×10^9 base-pairs (bp), and diploid cells contain twice that amount. Thus the potential information content of the human genome is enormous, far greater than is necessary to determine the upper limit of about 100 000 functional genes in the human genome. Most of this DNA has no known purpose. It is now customary to restrict the term gene to those parts of the genome that have a coding function, either by being transcribed into RNA or by being both transcribed into RNA and subsequently translated into protein. Also scattered through the genome are a number of pseudo-genes, DNA sequences that have the structure of expressed genes, and were presumably functional earlier in evolution, but which have

Table 3.1. *Bases, nucleosides and nucleotides*

Type	Base	Nucleoside	Nucleotide
Purine	Adenine	Adenosine	Adenylic acid
Purine	Guanine	Guanosine	Guanylic acid
Pyrimidine	Cytosine	Cytidine	Cytidylic acid
Pyrimidine	Thymine	Thymidine	Thymidylic acid
Pyrimidine	Uracil	Uridine	Uridylic acid

now acquired mutations rendering them incapable of producing a protein product.

TRANSCRIPTION OF DNA INTO RNA

The structure of RNA is similar to that of DNA, except that the sugar component of the backbone is ribose rather than deoxyribose, uracil (U) replaces thymine (T) and the molecule is single-stranded. Several different types of RNA are found in the cell. Both ribosomal RNA and transfer RNA are involved in protein synthesis, but the essential connecting link between the information contained in a gene and its end result as the amino acid sequence of a protein is messenger RNA (mRNA).

A simplified version of DNA transcription into mRNA is shown in Fig. 3.3. The 5' to 3' DNA strand is known as the sense or coding strand and the 3' to 5' DNA strand as the antisense or anticoding strand.* An enzyme, RNA polymerase II, using the double-stranded DNA molecule as template, produces a single-stranded mRNA molecule that is an exact copy of the sense DNA strand, apart from the substitution of U for T. In this way, the information content of the DNA molecule is maintained during transcription into an mRNA molecule, which, after processing, carries the information from the nucleus into the cytoplasm of the cell.

Closer inspection of RNA synthesis reveals a more complex picture. Most eukaryotic genes are interrupted by stretches of DNA that, although transcribed into RNA, are not translated into protein. These

---

* In some textbooks this convention is reversed on the grounds that RNA polymerase must use the 3' to 5' DNA strand as template, and therefore that DNA strand should be called the sense strand. However, RNA polymerase requires both DNA strands as template, and a convention in which the sense of RNA runs in the same direction as the sense of DNA is easier to remember.

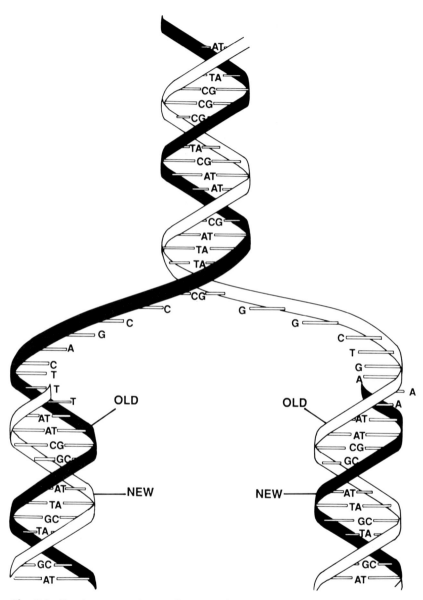

Fig. 3.2. Semi-conservative replication of DNA. Unwinding of the parental duplex provides templates for synthesis of new strands using the base-pairing rules. Each daughter duplex contains one old and one new strand.

are known as intervening sequences (IVS) or introns, whereas the translated sequences are known as exons. The size of most human genes is determined by the number and size of the introns; for example the β-globin gene is about 1600 bp in size, but only 438 bp are needed to code for the β-globin protein (Fig. 3.4). The recently discovered cystic fibrosis gene is about 250 000 bp (or 250 kilobase-pairs (kb)), whereas its protein product needs only 6500 bp of instruction. The muscular dystrophy gene is gigantic, more than 2500 kb in length, of which less than 1% is organized into exons.

When DNA is transcribed into RNA, the primary product (the mRNA precursor) contains both introns and exons. Introns are then spliced out in a process that depends on recognition sites at the beginning and end of the intron. Introns always begin with the dinucleotide GT (the splice donor) and end with AG (the splice acceptor): adjacent bases have limited variations within what is known as a consensus sequence. The mature mRNA thus contains

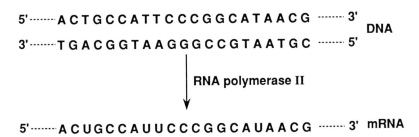

Fig. 3.3. Simplified model of DNA transcription. The enzyme RNA polymerase II produces an RNA copy of the 5' to 3' sense DNA strand, except that it substitutes U for T.

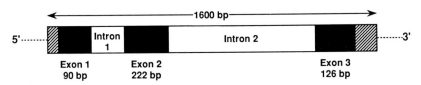

Fig. 3.4. Structure of the β-globin gene. Filled boxes represent exons, open boxes introns, and cross-hatched boxes represent untranslated regions at the 5' and 3' ends of the gene. Note that of the approximately 1600 bp of the gene only 438 bp are contained in exons.

the exon sequences of the sense DNA strand with the introns removed (Fig. 3.5).

A more detailed representation of DNA transcription is shown in Fig. 3.6. The enzyme RNA polymerase needs a signal to indicate a DNA sequence appropriate for transcription. This is provided by blocks of DNA at the 5′ end (i.e. upstream) of the gene, known as promoter sequences or regulatory boxes. The first of these, 20–30 bp upstream, is the TATA box, and another sequence 70–90 bp upstream is called the CCAAT box. These regions, together with other less well-defined sequences even further upstream, are responsible for the rate of DNA transcription into RNA and also, for some genes, the tissue-specific nature of the process. Transcription starts at the cap site, and the precursor mRNA is capped or blocked with 7-methyl-guanosine at its 5′ end. There follows a short untranslated region, the leader sequence, and then the initiation codon, ATG, which specifies the initiation of translation. A stop codon indicates the end of the translated region of the gene. However, both precursor and mature

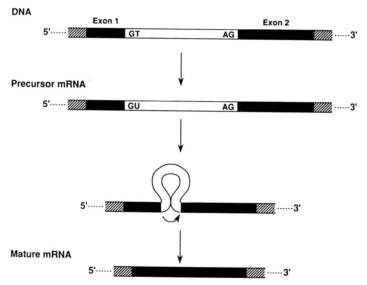

Fig. 3.5. Diagrammatic representation of the splicing out of an intron from precursor mRNA. The splice donor GT in DNA becomes GU in the precursor mRNA, whereas the splice acceptor AG is unchanged. Consensus nucleotides at the donor and acceptor sites are not shown. Sequences at the 5′ and 3′ ends of both DNA and RNA are explained more fully in Fig. 3.6.

mRNA have untranslated sequences at the 3' end that include a signal for the addition of a string of adenosine residues (poly(A)). The capping and tailing of RNA is probably necessary to permit its export from the nucleus. All these processes, together with the splicing out of introns, occur in the nucleus and the mature mRNA is now ready for export to the cytoplasm.

TRANSLATION OF RNA INTO PROTEIN

Once in the cytoplasm, mRNA functions as a template for the synthesis of proteins from their constituent amino acid residues. The exact mechanism of translation is complex and involves a family of transfer RNAs (tRNA), each of which carries a specific amino acid and which also has a specific 3 bp recognition site (the anticodon) for mRNA. Ribosomes, which are cytoplasmic organelles made of ribosomal RNA and protein, mediate translation by moving along the mRNA and allowing the anticodons of tRNA to recognize appropriate codons in mRNA (Fig. 3.7). The important feature of this process is that genetic information, originally coded in the exon sequences of the gene, is transferred through mRNA to the correct amino acid sequence in the growing polypeptide chain.

The correlation between bases in mRNA, and obviously also in the DNA from which the RNA was transcribed, and amino acid residues is known as the genetic code. It is a triplet code with 3-base sequences (codons) specifying particular amino acids (Table 3.2). Since there are 64 possible codons and only 20 unmodified amino acids found in

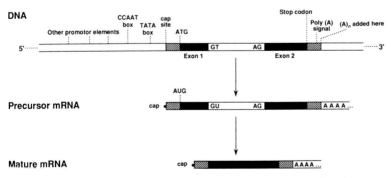

Fig. 3.6. A more complete representation of transcription showing the cap site and promotor elements at the 5' end and the poly(A) signal at the 3' end of the gene. Note that capping and tailing of precursor mRNA precede the splicing out of introns.

protein, the code is degenerate, and each amino acid, with the exception of methionine and tryptophan, has more than one codon. Many of the different codons for single amino acids differ only in the third nucleotide of the triplet. The RNA codons UAA, UAG and UGA (corresponding to TAA, TAG and TGA in DNA) lead to a termination of translation and are called stop or termination codons.

Protein synthesis proceeds along the mRNA template in the 5' to 3' direction. The growing polypeptide chain is synthesized from the amino-terminal end to the carboxyl-terminal end. In eukaryotic systems the first amino acid residue is always methionine (mRNA codon AUG), although this is often rapidly removed after incorporation into protein. For most proteins there follows a series of post-translational modifications, such as removal of leader sequences, glycosylation, phosphorylation or attachment of coenzymes. None the less, the amino acid sequence of the mature protein is determined by the exon structure of the gene that encodes it.

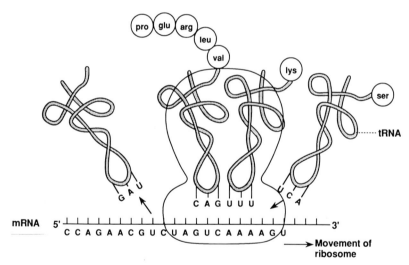

Fig. 3.7. Mechanism of translation of mRNA into protein. Each tRNA has an anticodon recognition site for codons in mRNA and carries a specific amino acid, e.g. the tRNA at the right carries serine and its anticodon UCA recognises the serine codon AGU. Amino acids attach serially to the growing polypeptide chain and the respective tRNAs are discharged (at left). The process is mediated by ribosomes (one is shown in outline) moving along the mRNA in a 5'→3' direction.

Table 3.2. *The genetic code*

RNA codons	Amino acid	Abbreviations[a]	
GCA, GCC, GCG, GCU	Alanine	ala	A
AGA, AGG, CGA, CGC, CGG, CGU	Arginine	arg	R
GAC, GAU	Aspartic acid	asp	D
AAC, AAU	Asparagine	asn	N
UGC, UGU	Cysteine	cys	C
GAA, GAG	Glutamic acid	glu	E
CAA, CAG	Glutamine	gln	Q
GGA, GGC, GGG, GGU	Glycine	gly	G
CAC, CAU	Histidine	his	H
AUA, AUC, AUU	Isoleucine	ile	I
UUA, UUG, CUA, CUC, CUG, CUU	Leucine	leu	L
AAA, AAG	Lysine	lys	K
AUG	Methionine	met	M
UUC, UUU	Phenylalanine	phe	F
CCA, CCC, CCG, CCU	Proline	pro	P
AGC, AGU, UCA, UCC, UCG, UCU	Serine	ser	S
ACA, ACC, ACG, ACU	Threonine	thr	T
UGG	Tryptophan	trp	W
UAC, UAU	Tyrosine	tyr	Y
GUA, GUC, GUG, GUU	Valine	val	V
UAA, UAG, UGA	Stop		

Note: [a]Three-letter and one-letter abbreviations.

BASIC TECHNIQUES OF DNA ANALYSIS

There is a very large amount of DNA in human cells. Each nucleated diploid cell contains some 2 m of DNA, made up of sequences containing about 6×10^9 to 7×10^9 pairs of nucleotides. The DNA is packaged into 46 chromosomes, the largest of which (no. 1) contains about 3×10^8 bp, whereas the smallest (no. 21) contains about 0.5×10^8 bp. Thus, even when a pure preparation of chromosome 21 is made, the constituent DNA is sufficient to code for about 16 000 genes of average length 3000 bp. Furthermore, the DNA in each chromosome is continuous and there are no obvious features to distinguish one gene from another.

The sheer size of native DNA coupled to its relative chemical homogeneity has, for many years, thwarted attempts to carry out genetic analysis in the obvious way – by the isolation and characterization of genes themselves. Recently, a number of quite complex techniques have evolved for the manipulation of DNA – a science often referred to as genetic engineering. In this chapter, I concentrate mainly on one facet of genetic engineering, the analysis and measurement of segments of DNA that often represent genes themselves or that can be used to track the segregation of genes in families. More advanced aspects of gene manipulation are covered in specialist books.

HYBRIDIZATION

When native double-stranded DNA is isolated, dissolved in solution and heated, the hydrogen bonds between base-pairs are weakened and eventually ruptured. The two strands begin to unwind and eventually separate from one another to give single-stranded DNA. The process, called denaturation, depends on the base composition of the DNA and on the pH and ionic strength of the solution. At low ionic strength, denaturation is quite sudden and there is a characteristic transition point called the melting temperature: this ranges from 80°C to 95°C for different natural DNAs. When the hot solution of single-stranded DNA is allowed to cool slowly, complementary strands gradually find each other and reassociate or anneal to the original double-stranded form.

The ability of denatured single-stranded DNA molecules to find complementary sequences to which they can anneal is the key to many forms of DNA analysis. If an exogenous single-stranded DNA molecule, with sequences complementary to the original DNA, is introduced into the hot solution and the solution allowed to cool slowly, there will be competition between the exogenous and original DNAs to form double-stranded sequences. Some hybrid double-stranded molecules will be formed, along with the original renatured DNA and also renatured exogenous DNA. Hybridization is favoured by a relatively high concentration of exogenous material, although this also produces an excess of double-stranded exogenous DNA.

Solution hybridization, sometimes called liquid hybridization, is not a suitable technique for investigating the complementarity of two different DNA preparations. Three different types of molecule result, and it is difficult to assess the proportions represented by the hybrid. This difficulty was overcome when it was discovered that certain types of inert support such as nitrocellulose or nylon filters would bind single-stranded DNA and prevent self-annealing, and yet still make the bound sequences available for hybridization to an exogenous single-stranded DNA. If the exogenous DNA, often referred to as a probe, was tagged with a radioactive label, the extent of hybridization could be assessed by measuring the amount of radio-activity that remained bound to the filter-immobilized DNA after careful washing (Fig. 3.8). Clearly, there will also be some self-reasso-ciation of the probe DNA, but this will be removed in the washing process. Filter hybridization is one of the most important analytical techniques currently used in gene analysis.

PROBES

To make DNA–DNA hybridization into a useful analytical technique it is necessary for the exogenous probe DNA to have some definable properties, and also to be recognizable by virtue of an easily detected tag, such as a radioactive or other marker. Three different types of DNA probe are widely used in gene analysis (Table 3.3).

Genomic DNA probes

These are segments of native double-stranded DNA that have been isolated and then amplified to high copy number by cloning in a

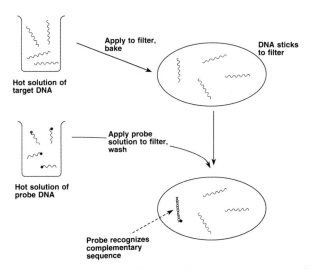

Fiq. 3.8. Principle of filter hybridization. Target double-stranded DNA is rendered single-stranded by heating, then applied to a nitrocellulose or nylon filter and baked. The filter is immersed in a solution of radiolabelled probe DNA, also rendered single-stranded by heating. Probe DNA hybridizes only to complementary sequences, and the hybrids may be detected by overlaying the filter with X-ray film.

37

Table 3.3. *Types of DNA probe*

Probe	Characteristics
Genomic probe	Amplified sequence of genomic DNA. Not usually an expressed gene. Often an anonymous sequence. Double-stranded
cDNA probe	Amplified sequence representing the exons of an expressed gene. Double or single-stranded
Oligonucleotide	Probe made up of a short sequence of nucleotides. Single-stranded

suitable vector. The technology of DNA cloning is complex and continues to evolve as more sophisticated vectors are developed that will carry larger and larger sequences of DNA. The simplest, and still widely used, vectors are plasmids. These are autonomous elements found in bacterial cells; their genomes can replicate in the cell independently of the host's chromosomal machinery. They are circular DNA molecules and often exist as multiple copies within the host cell. Since bacterial cells such as *Escherichia coli* can be grown rapidly in laboratory culture, plasmid DNA can also be amplified vastly in a matter of a few days.

One of the fundamental tricks of recombinant DNA technology is the ability to insert a segment of human genomic DNA into a circular plasmid and then to grow up the hybrid plasmid–human material in a host cell. The strategy is illustrated in Fig. 3.9 for the much used plasmid vector pBR322. The first step is to isolate the plasmid from its *E. coli* host and to cut it open with a suitable restriction endonuclease (described in detail below). The human genomic DNA required as a probe is introduced into the linearized plasmid and the hybrid plasmid recircularized. It can now be re-introduced into the host *E. coli*. A useful trick is to use a plasmid that contains two different antibiotic resistance genes. One of these, e.g. ampicillin resistance (Ap^R) can be used to distinguish transformed *E. coli* cells (those that have taken up plasmid) from untransformed cells. The other, e.g. tetracycline resistance (Tc^R), can be arranged in such a way that it is destroyed by the introduction into the plasmid of the human DNA. In this way, the three classes of *E. coli* can be distinguished – untrans-

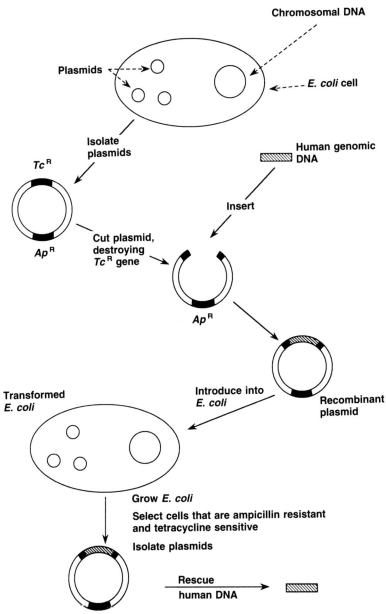

Fig. 3.9. A strategy for cloning human genomic DNA. See the text for details. The amplification of human DNA depends both on the growth of E. *coli* cells and on the independent multiplication of recombinant plasmids in the E. *coli* cells.

formed cells (no plasmid) are sensitive to both ampicillin and tetra-cycline, while *E. coli* transformed by the hybrid plasmid is resistant to ampicillin but sensitive to tetracycline. Once the desired type of *E. coli* has been grown up, the hybrid plasmid can be isolated and the human DNA rescued. In this way, considerable quantities of purified genomic DNA can be prepared, ready for tagging with a radioactive marker.

The most useful genomic DNA probes are those that correspond to the whole or part of a defined gene. Obviously, such gene probes, when rendered single-stranded will seek out and hybridize to that stretch of DNA in the genome that represents the gene or some part of it. However, most genomic probes in current usage are anonymous, so termed because they represent stretches of DNA of unknown function. Many have been produced by cloning DNA from defined regions of specific chromosomes, so that their anonymity is qualified by an approximate indication of their position in the human genome. Their usefulness is generally established by their proximity to a disease-causing gene, a tedious and time-consuming process that will be described later. Anonymous probes are first given in-house names that have significance only to the laboratory from which they originated. Once their chromosomal location is established, they are assigned to a letter and numbering system, e.g. D4S23 is a DNA segment on chromosome 4 and was the 23rd to be registered.

Complementary DNA (cDNA) probes
The sequence of bases in genomic DNA contains a great deal more information than is needed to code for the amino acid sequence in its protein product. In contrast, mature mRNA, from which intervening sequences have been removed by normal cellular processing (Fig. 3.5), is complementary to the essential exon sequences of the gene. Enzymes known as reverse transcriptases are able to use mRNA as a template to produce complementary DNA (or cDNA) copies of the exon structures of the genes from which they are derived.

One strategy for making cDNA probes is to isolate mRNA from a tissue in which it is particularly abundant. For example, reticulocyte mRNA is made up largely of species encoding the α- and β-globin proteins. The mRNA can be reverse transcribed (using a short syn-thetic primer to start the reaction) into a single-stranded DNA mol-ecule that is exactly complementary (Fig. 3.10). The RNA molecule is removed by alkaline degradation or by a ribonuclease (RNase) enzyme and the single-stranded cDNA rendered double-stranded by another round of reverse transcription or by use of a bacterial DNA polymerase. The resulting double-stranded cDNA molecules can then be cloned into plasmids and amplified to high copy number.

Oligonucleotide probes

Genomic and cDNA probes are relatively large molecules that can be complementary to the whole or a significant part of a gene. In contrast, oligonucleotides are short stretches of DNA, conventionally 17 to 25 bases in length, that have been synthesized by a chemical reaction in which each base is added sequentially to the preceding one. Their composition can be defined exactly and oligonucleotides of any required base sequence can be constructed. Because these probes are synthetic and can be made in reasonable quantity on automatic DNA synthesizers, there is no need to resort to bacterial amplification systems to obtain adequate amounts of reagent. Furthermore, they are single-stranded, and thus ready to hybridize to complementary single-stranded targets.

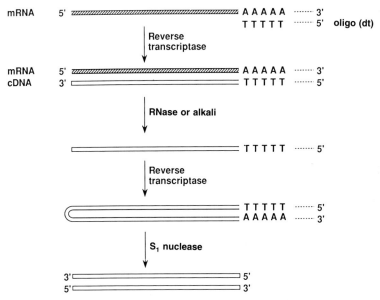

Fig. 3.10. Preparation of a cDNA probe by reverse transcription. The first step uses mRNA as template and a short oligo(dT) primer for synthesis of cDNA by reverse transcriptase. The RNA is removed by RNase or alkaline hydrolysis. The single-stranded cDNA serves as its own primer and template for second-strand synthesis by reverse transcriptase, after which the hairpin loop is removed using a single-strand-specific nuclease.

41

At first sight, it might seem surprising that a 17 base oli-gonucleotide (referred to as a 17-mer) should have the specificity to recognize only one sequence of genomic DNA. However, the number of different ways in which four different bases can be arranged in a 17 base sequence is very large – 4^{17} or about 17×10^9. The haploid human genome contains about 3.5×10^9 bp, so it is probable that any defined 17 base sequence will not be repeated more than at most a few times in the genome. To ensure that an oligonucleotide will hybridize to only an exactly complementary sequence in the genome and not to any closely analogous sequence, oligonucleotide hybridization is usu-ally carried out under conditions of high stringency; that is at temperatures and in solutions of ionic strength that favour the forma-tion of exact duplexes.

One of the principal advantages of oligonucleotide probes is that they have the specificity to recognize a single-base alteration in the sequence to which they are directed. Many genetic disorders are the consequence of point mutations in the gene, in which the normal nucleotide has been substituted by an incorrect nucleotide. Genomic and cDNA probes, which may be several thousand bases in length, cannot detect such subtle changes and will hybridize to the normal and mutant gene with equal affinity. Under the right conditions of sufficient stringency, an oligonucleotide will base-pair with only the exactly complementary sequence and not with a sequence that differs by a single base (Fig. 3.11). It is usual practice to use oligonucleotides

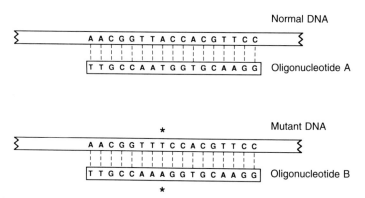

Fig. 3.11. A 17 bp oligonucleotide A hybridizes to a complementary sequence in normal DNA, but the single base-pair difference in the mutant DNA (asterisk) prevents recognition. Oligonucleotide B, complementary to the mutant sequence, hybridizes to mutant but not to normal DNA.

in pairs, one member designed to be complementary to the normal sequence and the other complementary to the mutant sequence. This provides the type of control necessary to ensure that hybridization or non-hybridization is not the result of incorrect conditions.

RESTRICTION ENZYMES

The genomic DNA of mammalian cells consists of very large molecules, and tends to be broken by mechanical shearing during the isolation process. The resulting preparation has fragments of varying sizes, but since shearing is semi-random there is no way of ensuring that a particular DNA sequence is contained in any given fragment size. Furthermore, different preparations from the same source may give different sets of DNA fragments if the conditions of isolation vary even slightly.

The resolution of this impasse came from the discovery in the early 1970s of bacterial enzymes that have the property of cleaving DNA in a highly specific manner. The most important of these restriction endonucleases (often referred to as restriction enzymes) translocate along double-stranded DNA until they find a particular sequence of bases that constitutes the recognition or cleavage site. At this site, and no other, they cleave both strands of the DNA. The most common recognition sites are sequences of four or six bases, but some restriction endonucleases require a sequence of five, seven, eight or even more bases. Many recognition sites have an axis of symmetry and are said to be palindromic, meaning that the sequence in the coding strand read backwards gives the sequence in the anticoding strand (Fig. 3.12). The axis of symmetry does not necessarily mean that cleavage has to give an even break with flush ends (as occurs with *Hae*II and *Hpa*I). Cleavage more often produces termini with short single-stranded ends known as cohesive or sticky ends (e.g. *Taq*I, *Eco*RI).

On average, a restriction enzyme recognizing a four-base sequence will find a target every 4^4 (256) bases in a random DNA sequence. A six base cutter will find a target every 4^6 (4096) bases. Thus, enzymes such as *Taq*I and *Hae*III will tend to produce smaller DNA fragments than those produced by *Eco*RI or *Hpa*I. Some enzymes recognize sequences with a degree of ambiguity: *Hind*II accepts either C or T in the third base and either A or G in the fourth base of its hexanucleotide recognition sequence, and the site is designated $CT(^C_T)(^A_G)$ AC or CTPyPuAC (C and T are pyrimidines (Py), A and G are purines (Pu)). Others are even less fussy and any nucleotide in a particular position will do: e.g. *Hinf*I accepts GANTC where N can be A, C, G or T.

Over 1000 different restriction enzymes are now known, a large proportion of which are commercially available. They are named after the parent organism from which they are isolated and, if necessary, the strain or serotype and chronological order of isolation. Thus *Hinf*I was the first restriction enzyme to be isolated from *Haemophilus*

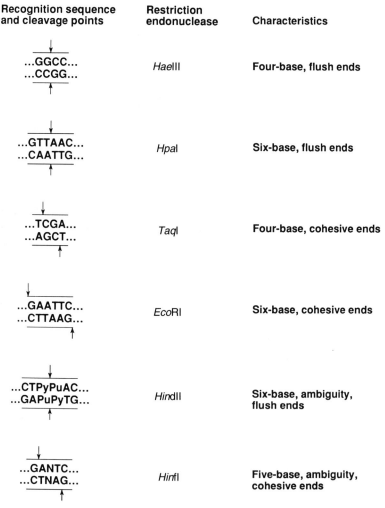

Recognition sequence and cleavage points	Restriction endonuclease	Characteristics
...GGCC... ...CCGG...	*Hae*III	Four-base, flush ends
...GTTAAC... ...CAATTG...	*Hpa*I	Six-base, flush ends
...TCGA... ...AGCT...	*Taq*I	Four-base, cohesive ends
...GAATTC... ...CTTAAG...	*Eco*RI	Six-base, cohesive ends
...CTPyPuAC... ...GAPuPyTG...	*Hind*II	Six-base, ambiguity, flush ends
...GANTC... ...CTNAG...	*Hinf*I	Five-base, ambiguity, cohesive ends

Fig. 3.12. Characteristics of some restriction enzymes. Py, pyrimidine (C, T); Pu, purine (A, G); N, any nucleotide.

influenzae strain f, and *Hind*II the second to be isolated from *Haemophilus influenzae* strain d. Laboratory pronunciation attempts to make easy words of the abbreviations; *Hae*III becomes hay three, *Taq*I becomes tack one, and so on.

The most remarkable feature of restriction enzymes is their specificity, the ability to cut DNA only when the right recognition site is seen. Different digestions of the same DNA sample will in principle, and usually in practice (if conditions are kept constant), give an identical set of restriction fragments. If a four- or six-base-specific enzyme is used, the molecular size of the fragments will usually be in the range where they can be manipulated and separated from each other by electrophoresis on an agarose gel. In a simple organism such as bacteriophage λ, digestion of genomic DNA with *Eco*RI gives a set of only six or seven restriction fragments that can be separated on an agarose gel and visualized by staining with ethidium bromide. However, in more complex organisms such as humans, the large genome size leads to a vast array of fragments and gel electrophoresis shows a continuous smear of bands. In these cases other methods must be used to identify individual fragments.

SOUTHERN BLOTTING

Restriction endonuclease cleavage enables high molecular weight native DNA to be cut in a reproducible fashion into a set of fragments of more manageable size. Hybridization to a tagged probe provides a mechanism for identifying specific sequences within the set of fragments. However, to turn these two procedures into a robust analytical tool that would give a physical position to the fragment of interest, further manipulation was needed. This came through the description by Ed Southern in 1975 of a procedure of such wide applicability that it has come to bear his name. Southern blotting is outlined in Fig. 3.13 and the component steps described in more detail below.

Extraction and digestion

Double-stranded genomic DNA can be extracted quite readily from any source of nucleated cells. The most frequently used tissues for human gene analysis are the white cell fraction of blood and the cells of a chorionic villus biopsy. DNA is solubilized, protein and other impurities removed by extraction with a chloroform–phenol mixture, and the DNA precipitated using ethanol and re-solubilized in an appropriate buffer. The yield can be monitored in an ultraviolet spectrophotometer. A 20 ml blood sample should give about 200 μg DNA and a 50 mg chorionic villus biopsy about 50 μg DNA.

A sample of DNA, conventionally 5 µg to 10 µg, is then incubated with the restriction enzyme of choice. Completeness of digestion can be monitored by removing a small sample of the mix and running it out electrophoretically on an agarose gel. Native DNA is of too high a molecular weight to penetrate far into the gel, while fully digested DNA will spread into the gel and can be visualized after ethidium-bromide staining under ultraviolet light.

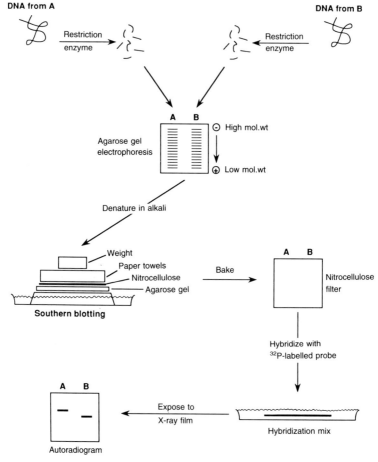

Fig. 3.13. A schematic representation of Southern blotting. See the text for details.

Gel electrophoresis

The whole digested sample is subjected to horizontal electrophoresis on an agarose gel. Fragments are separated on the basis of molecular size, with low molecular weight components migrating more rapidly towards the anode. In contrast to protein electrophoresis, all DNA fragments are negatively charged and move in the same direction from the origin of application. A size marker, often a restricted preparation of DNA from bacteriophage λ that contains a set of six or seven fragments of known molecular size, is run simultaneously in a separate slot on the gel, and provides a reference for subsequent size calibrations.

Transfer to a filter

The suspended DNA fragments on the agarose gel are double-stranded. In order to allow them to attach to a nitrocellulose or nylon filter they must be denatured and made single-stranded. This is usually achieved by soaking in a strong alkaline solution prior to transfer. For nitrocellulose blots, the gel must be neutralized in a strong buffer solution before transfer.

In classical Southern blotting, single-stranded DNA in the agarose gel is transferred to the filter by placing a stack of dry paper towels at the top of a sandwich formed by the agarose gel at the bottom and a nitrocellulose or nylon sheet in the middle. The gel is kept moist by placing it on a thick layer of filter paper dipping into a suitable buffer. Single-stranded DNA is carried by the flow of buffer from gel to filter and is trapped there. Once transfer is complete, the filter is baked to immobilize the trapped DNA. In theory, and usually in practice, the filter carries a perfect single-stranded replica of the original double-stranded DNA separated by electrophoresis on the agarose gel.

DNA samples can also be transferred from an agarose gel to the filter using vacuum blotting. Instead of using a stack of dry paper towels to facilitate solution movement, the filter is fitted exactly to the gel and the top surface subjected to a mild vacuum. Transfer of DNA from the gel to the filter is more rapid in this method, but may not be as complete for the high molecular weight fragments. A specially constructed vacuum apparatus is necessary.

Hybridization

The baked filter is first prehybridized to saturate the vacant filter sites with an inert DNA and thus to avoid background binding of the tagged probe. The filter is then hybridized by incubating with the

47

radioactive probe, rendered single-stranded by a rapid boiling and quenching step. The exact conditions of hybridization depend on the nature of the target DNA and the characteristics of probe DNA, but are often carried out at a temperature of around 65°C for a period of 12 to 18 hours. Once hybridization is complete, the filter is washed in a series of buffer solutions to remove excess probe DNA. The exact composition of wash buffers and the temperature of washing influences the degree of binding of probe to target DNA, and is established by empirical variation of established protocols.

Autoradiography and other forms of visualization
The final step in Southern blotting is to identify regions of the filter to which the probe has bound. In most cases the probe has been labelled with ^{32}P and binding is revealed by autoradiography. The filter is placed in a metal cassette, overlayed with X-ray film and left at -70°C for several days. After development of the film, bound DNA shows up as darkened bands on a light background. If the probe has been labelled with a non-radioisotopic marker, its binding position on the filter must be determined by other methods.

THE SIGNIFICANCE OF SOUTHERN BLOTTING
As illustrated in Fig. 3.13, Southern blotting enables a particular sequence of bases in the midst of a large jumble of DNA fragments to be identified by hybridization to an appropriate probe and detection by autoradiography or other non-isotopic methods. In considering the uses to which Southern blotting may be put, it is important to note a critical point about hybridization. A genomic or cDNA probe will hybridize to target DNA to which it is complementary; however, if the target DNA is cut by a restriction enzyme into a number of fragments of reasonable molecular size, the probe will now identify each of these fragments at a different site on the Southern blot (Fig. 3.14). Even though the probe contains some sequences that are not used in hybridizing to the target fragments, those sequences that do hybridize are still fully complementary. Likewise, the probe will hybridize satisfactorily to fragments of DNA that it covers only partly, e.g. the fragment of 2.5 kb shown in Fig. 3.14.

For the past ten years, Southern blotting has been the foundation stone of gene analysis in inherited diseases. It is most frequently used to make comparisons between the genetic make-up of different individuals, the DNA from the different samples being digested with the same restriction enzyme and the blot hybridized with the same probe. This is most easily visualized by considering the detection of a gene deletion in a disorder inherited as autosomal recessive.

The prime example is the South-east Asian variety of α-thalassaemia, a condition leading to hydrops fetalis and intrauterine death. In some cases of this disorder there is an extensive deletion of both α-globin genes from the 30 kb cluster on chromosome 16, which also contains a functional ζ-gene (Fig. 3.15). The α-globin region may be isolated by digesting genomic DNA with the restriction enzyme *Bgl*II, which, by cutting at three sites near the α-globin genes, generates two unequal-sized fragments complementary to an α-globin probe. In normal individuals and in those heterozygous for the deletion, a Southern blot shows bands at 12.6 kb and at 7.4 kb. In the homozygous affected individual neither fragment is present. It should be noted that, in principle, it is possible to distinguish a heterozygote from a normal homozygote by virtue of diminished intensity of the bands. In practice, Southern blot band intensities are used for the measurement of gene copy number only under carefully controlled conditions.

Restriction sites and fragment sizes

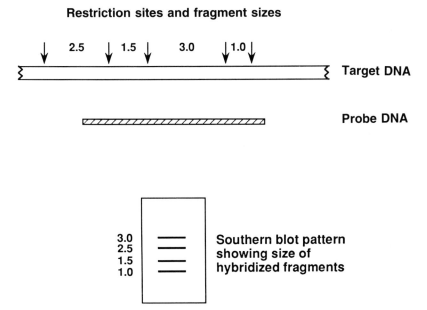

Fig. 3.14. Scheme indicating how a single DNA probe may hybridize to several different fragments of target DNA after Southern blotting.

The example of Southern blotting to detect the deletion of a gene or group of genes is the most obvious use of this powerful method of DNA analysis. As is shown in later chapters, Southern blots can distinguish much more subtle gene alterations, including single-base changes in a sequence of many thousands of bases. The principle that needs to be emphasized is that this technique is always used to make comparisons of gene structure, either between individuals in a family in which a genetic disease is segregating or between unrelated individuals who may vary in some important aspect of their genomic constitution.

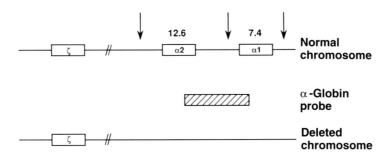

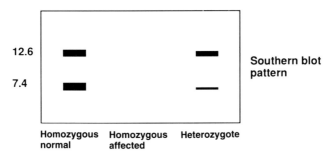

Fig. 3.15. Use of Southern blotting to detect a gene deletion in α-thalassaemia. On the normal chromosome, *Bgl*II generates fragments of sizes 12.6 and 7.4 kb that hybridize to an α-globin gene probe. These fragments are absent from the deleted chromosome. In principle it is possible to distinguish heterozygotes from normal homozygotes; in practice this is difficult.

DOT (SLOT) BLOTTING

In some circumstances it is not necessary to separate digested DNA by gel electrophoresis prior to hybridization to a probe. The DNA can be spotted directly onto a filter as a series of dots (or slots), each dot representing a different sample or a different dilution of the same sample. Obviously genomic DNA must be rendered single-stranded before it will bind to the filter, and viscous high molecular weight

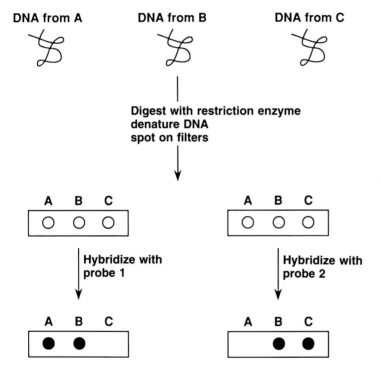

A has gene corresponding to probe 1
C has gene corresponding to probe 2
B has genes corresponding to probe 1 and probe 2

Fig. 3.16. The use of dot blotting to compare DNA from three different individuals. In this example, A is homozygous for sequences complementary to probe 1 and C homozygous for sequences complementary to probe 2. B is a heterozygote with sequences complementary to both probes.

DNA is usually reduced in size by sonication or restriction enzyme digestion prior to application.

The material in dot blots contains all the original DNA in the preparation. Hybridization is therefore carried out under conditions of high stringency to avoid spurious reactions between the probe and non-complementary sequences. Genomic and cDNA probes may be used in dot blotting to detect major changes in the genomic material, such as the presence or absence of Y-chromosome sequences, which would distinguish male and female fetuses. However, most applications of dot blotting employ pairs of oligonucleotide probes, with the ability to recognize DNA sequences differing by only a single base-pair (Fig. 3.16).

THE POLYMERASE CHAIN REACTION

Most genes of interest in medical genetics are present as a single copy, or, at most, as a few copies, in the human genome. Thus if 10μg of DNA were used as the starting point for Southern or dot-blotting analysis, the amount of a specific gene to be detected might be as little as 10^{-5} μg. Even when the hybridizing probe is labelled with radioactive phosphorus to maximum specific activity it may take up to a week of exposure to X-ray film before specific bands can be visualized. Biotin-labelled probes are in general no more sensitive, so most laboratories continue to use worryingly large amounts of potentially hazardous radiolabel.

In 1985, a powerful new procedure was reported that allows selected regions of the genome to be amplified by a factor of 10^6 or more in an in vitro reaction. The polymerase chain reaction (PCR) is simple in both concept and execution, but depends on knowledge of the exact DNA sequence of at least part of the region being amplified. In essence it is a series of three-step cycles, with the cycles being repeated 20 to 30 times to give an exponential increase of product. At 100% efficiency in each cycle, a double-stranded DNA segment will yield 2^{20} ($>10^6$) copies after 20 cycles and 2^{30} ($>10^9$) copies after 30 cycles. In practice, efficiencies are less than 100%, but it is still comparatively easy to produce 10^6 to 10^8 copies of a DNA segment in a few hours.

The outline of the PCR is shown in Fig. 3.17. The essential requirement is a pair of oligonucleotides, called primers, complementary to sequences at the ends of the double-stranded DNA to be amplified. Primers can be as short as 12 bp or as long as 50 bp, but obviously these particular sequences of the target DNA must be known exactly. One primer is complementary to a selected end of the coding or sense strand and the other primer complementary to a selected end of the

52

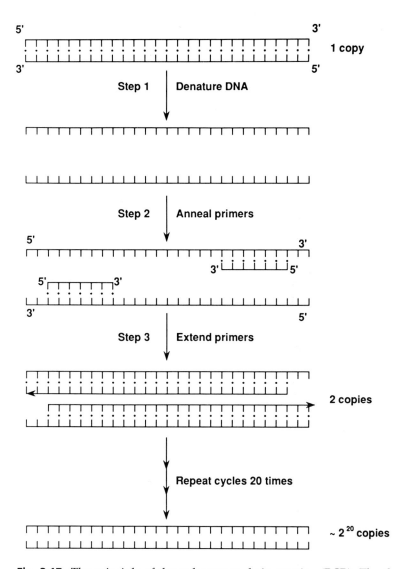

Fig. 3.17. The principle of the polymerase chain reaction (PCR). The three steps in the cycle are denaturation of double-stranded DNA, annealing of primers to opposite ends of the target region and extension of the primers with a DNA polymerase. Repetition of the cycle generates copies of the DNA between the primers in an exponential manner.

53

THE TECHNOLOGY OF MOLECULAR GENETICS

antisense strand; the region that is amplified lies between these selected ends. Sequences of up to several kilobases have been amplified by the PCR; on occasion, the sequence of the region between the primers has not been known.

The first step in the PCR is a short heat treatment that denatures the double-stranded target DNA. In the second step, the sample is cooled briefly to allow the primers to anneal to their respective separated strands. Primers are used in very large molar excess ($>10^8$), since they drive the reaction. In the third step, a DNA polymerase uses added nucleotide bases to extend the primers in opposite directions with the target DNA serving as template. At the completion of the first cycle of three steps there are now two copies of the target DNA, or four strands, with each strand able to serve as a template for the next PCR cycle.

Closer inspection of the mechanics of the PCR shows that in the first few cycles the product is heterogeneous in length, since there is no natural stopping point for primer extension. Correct-length copies appear at the end of the second cycle and double with each subsequent cycle, while incorrect-length copies increase only additively. By the end of the fourth cycle, correct-length copies are in a majority and their proportion increases with each subsequent cycle.

When the PCR was first introduced it was a rather tedious technique, since fresh DNA polymerase had to be added after each heat-denaturation step. The isolation of a thermostable DNA polymerase from the bacterium *Thermus aquaticus* (*Taq*) has greatly improved the performance of the procedure. *Taq* polymerase retains its activity through the heat-denaturation step and does not need to be replaced after each cycle. Furthermore, the high temperature optimum of this enzyme increases significantly the specificity and yield of the PCR and allows much longer target sequences to be amplified. A genetically engineered *Taq* polymerase is now commercially available.

PCR has turned out to be so valuable in gene analysis that it must now be regarded as one of the basic techniques of DNA manipulation. It has three immediate advantages.

1 Specific sequences can be amplified from minute samples of DNA, not ordinarily amenable to analysis. These include blood spots, buccal cell scrapings, hair root bulbs and even single cells dissected from an eight-cell blastocyst prior to implantation. The PCR can be made even more sensitive and specific by use of a nested primer variation (Fig. 3.18). In this technique, an intermediate amplified product is

54

created by a series of PCR cycles, and then a final product is produced by using new primers nested between the original primers. This essentially removes unwanted background amplifications and allows the second set of PCR cycles to be applied to a more specific target.

2 The considerable amplification of target sequences in the original DNA makes product identification much easier. Hybridization of probes to a PCR-amplified DNA will, in general, give clearer patterns than hybridization to non-amplified DNA. However, it is often possible to detect product without any hybridization at all, since the amplified material is the dominant DNA species in the mixture. This is illustrated in Fig 3.19, where PCR amplification of exon 10 of the cystic fibrosis gene reveals the 3 bp deletion of the classical mutant by its migration

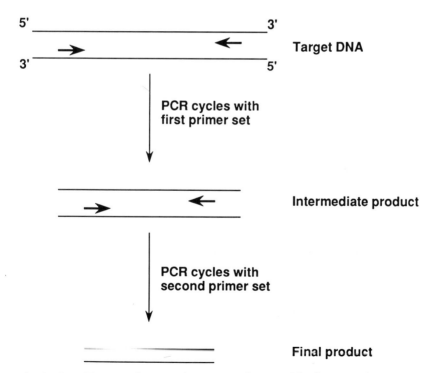

Fig. 3.18. PCR using the nested-primer technique. The first set of primers is used to produce an intermediate product, which is then used as the target material for the second set of primers.

position on an acrylamide gel. Amplification of exon 10 from normal individuals generates a 98 bp fragment, while amplification of exon 10 from homozygous affecteds generates a smaller and faster-moving 95 bp fragment. In individuals heterozygous for the classical cystic fibrosis mutation, known as ΔF_{508}, both 98 bp and 95 bp fragments, as well as characteristic heteroduplex fragments, are generated.

3 Since the PCR is, effectively, in vitro cloning, it can be used for the determination of the exact DNA sequence between the primers, without the usual cumbersome and time-consuming manipulations. This facet of the PCR will be discussed later.

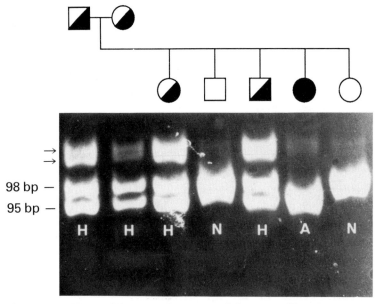

Fig. 3.19. PCR amplification of exon 10 of the cystic fibrosis gene and examination of products on an acrylamide gel. N, normal homozygote (98 bp fragment); A, affected homozygote (95 bp fragment); H, heterozygote. Note the characteristic heteroduplex fragments (arrows) in the samples from heterozygotes. Squares represent males, circles represent females.

MORE ADVANCED TECHNIQUES
MUTATIONAL ANALYSIS

Many X-linked and autosomal dominant disorders are associated with a high incidence of new mutations. In an X-linked recessive lethal, where all males died before passing on their mutant allele, the theoretical estimate of new mutations is one in three. In these disorders, of which Duchenne muscular dystrophy is the best example, there may be no prior knowledge of the exact nature of the mutant allele, except that it has occurred somewhere at the particular locus. Thus, in confirming the diagnosis of the disorder and in searching for the same mutation in other members of the family, it is often necessary to apply quite sophisticated methods of mutation analysis. Characterizing the mutant allele becomes an essential part of diagnosis, carrier detection and prenatal diagnosis.

In most recessively inherited disorders, new mutations are quite rare. However, virtually all genetic diseases are characterized by considerable heterogeneity, so that, at the DNA level, a named disorder is made up of a set of different mutant alleles. In some situations the laboratory investigator will have prior knowledge of which allele or combination of alleles is most likely to be segregating in the family or population at risk and will know how to carry out the appropriate analysis. In other situations the disorder may be caused by an as yet uncharacterized mutant allele and will therefore also need mutation analysis before exact methods of diagnosis can be applied.

The different ways in which unknown mutations can be detected fall into three broad groups:

1 Searching for major deletions or rearrangements.
2 Scanning for the approximate site of smaller mutations.
3 Defining the exact site and nature of the nucleotide alterations by sequencing methods.

Ultimately the precise delineation of any mutant allele always depends on DNA sequencing, but in cases of major deletions and re-arrangements such fine detail is often not essential.

Major deletions and rearrangements

It has already been pointed out that Southern blotting can be used to detect the α-globin gene deletions characteristic of the South-east Asian variety of α-thalassaemia (Fig. 3.15). However, this is a comparatively small genomic region, with both α-globin genes contained in about 20 kb of DNA, a size suitable for agarose gel electrophoresis.

In contrast, the dystrophin gene spans some 2500 kb, while the cystic fibrosis gene is 250 kb. Large genes can, of course, be cleaved into multiple small fragments of 20 kb or less, and each fragment then separated on an agarose gel, blotted and hybridized to an appropriate genomic or cDNA probe. This is a somewhat tedious process requiring multiple hybridizations to a panel of probes spanning as much of the gene as possible. It makes more sense to try to resolve genes as comparatively large fragments.

The difficulty here is that segments of DNA larger than about 50 kb all electro-migrate through agarose gels at about the same rate. They are no longer sieved by the pores of the gel but move end-on in a process known as reptation. One way of solving this problem is to

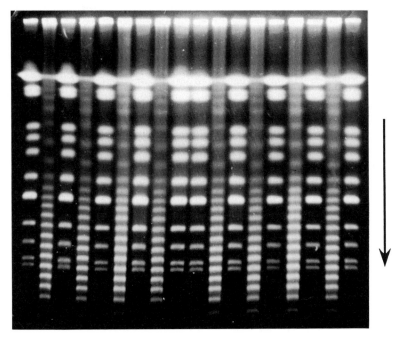

1 2 3 4 5 6 7 8 9 9 10 11 12 13 14 15 16 17

Fig. 3.20. Pulsed-field gel electrophoretic separation of large DNA fragments. The even-numbered lanes contain a ladder of molecular markers increasing in size (from the bottom of the gel) by multiples of 48.5 kb (e.g. 48.5, 97, 145.5, 194 kb etc.). The odd-numbered lanes contain a mixture of yeast chromosomes of sizes (from the bottom) 245, 280, 360, 450, 590, 680, 750, 790, 820, 940 and 970 kb. Courtesy of Dr Rakesh Anand.

use a technique called pulsed-field gel electrophoresis (PFGE), in which the DNA molecules are subjected alternately to two approximately perpendicular electric fields. When the direction of the field is switched, the DNA molecules re-orient themselves along the new field; large molecules take longer than small molecules both to do this and to re-align themselves when the direction of the field is switched back. The net effect of such field switching is a separation based on molecular size for fragments from 50 kb to about 1000 kb (Fig. 3.20). Several variations of PFGE have been described; one that is finding increasing favour is called field-inversion gel electrophoresis (FIGE). This is based on a uniform electric field but uses polarity switching in pulses (with longer forward than reverse pulses) to achieve separation.

Most commonly used restriction enzymes cut DNA into fairly small fragments, since their recognition sites occur frequently in the genome. Very large DNA fragments can be generated by *rare-cutters*, enzymes such as *Not*I, *Xho*I or *Sfi*I, whose cleavage sites are infrequent. These fragments, after PFGE or FIGE separation, can be either viewed directly with ethidium-bromide staining or blotted and hybridized to genomic or cDNA probes.

The PFGE/FIGE procedures are useful in analysing deletions in large genes and in mapping chromosomal rearrangements. They are of immediate practical diagnostic value in detecting possible carriers of the Duchenne muscular dystrophy gene. Such carriers have both a normal gene and a mutant gene, and in conventional Southern blotting it is often difficult to distinguish a diminished hybridization signal in a complex mixture of bands. If the carrier's DNA is fractionated with a rare-cutter restriction enzyme and resolved into a small set of well-separated PFGE-FIGE fragments, it is often possible to detect a new band that signals the presence of the mutant gene.

Scanning for smaller mutations

Many human genetic diseases are caused by point mutations, the alteration of a single base-pair in the DNA. A number of methods have evolved for the detection of such mutations (Table 3.4). All are scanning procedures in that they indicate the approximate site of the mutation, which must then be exactly delineated by DNA sequencing. Some, such as denaturing gradient gel electrophoresis are technically quite difficult and require special apparatus, while others, such as RNase A cleavage, do not detect all base-pair alterations. One of the most promising methods is chemical cleavage of mismatch (CCM) analysis outlined below.

Table 3.4. *Scanning methods for detection of point mutations*

Method	% of mutations detected
Denaturing gradient gel electrophoresis (DGGE)	50–100
RNase A cleavage	60–70
Single-strand conformation polymorphism analysis (SSCP)	Probably 100
Chemical cleavage of mismatch analysis (CCM)	Probably 100

The CCM method depends on the fact that if normal DNA is hybridized to a mutant DNA differing by a single base, the resulting heteroduplex will have a mismatched base-pair. If one of the mismatched bases is cytosine (C) it can be chemically modified by hydroxylamine, and if it is thymidine (T) it can be modified by osmium tetroxide. The use of these two reagents has given rise to the name HOT (hydroxylamine, osmium tetroxide) technique. After base modification, the particular DNA strand can be cleaved at that point by piperidine, and the fragments run out on a denaturing polyacrylamide gel. If the normal DNA has been radiolabelled prior to the reaction, the fragment sizes can be estimated by autoradiography and the approximate position of the mutation established (Fig. 3.21).

Several modifications to CCM have increased its power. The PCR can be used to generate adequate amounts of both normal and mutant DNA. If both strands of the normal DNA are radiolabelled in the PCR, guanosine (G) and adenosine (A) mismatches in the sense strand (not cleavable) will correspond to C and T mismatches in the antisense strand (cleavable). Thus, by using both strands of the normal DNA as probes, all possible base mismatches are detectable. Furthermore, it is claimed that small insertions and deletions can also be detected because they distort adjacent structures and even render base-paired C residues or T residues prone to reaction with hydroxylamine or osmium tetroxide.

Sequencing DNA

The ultimate definition of a mutation, often detected initially through a deletion or by a scanning method, is in determining the exact

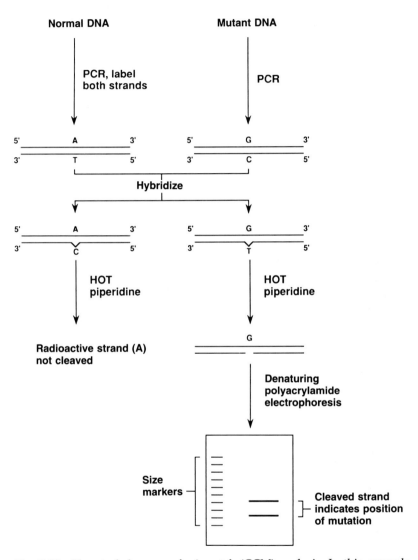

Fig. 3.21. Chemical cleavage of mismatch (CCM) analysis. In this example, mutant DNA differs from normal DNA by a single base-pair. In the resulting heteroduplexes, mismatched strands are cleaved, but only the cleaved radioactive strand (marked by T) is visualized on this schematic autoradiogram of the polyacrylamide gel.

alteration in the nucleotide sequence. There are two different methods of DNA sequence analysis, both depending on the power of polyacrylamide gels to resolve nucleic acid fragments differing in length by a single base. Although the method of Maxam and Gilbert, which employs chemical reagents to effect base-specific cleavage, is still widely used, it is gradually being displaced by dideoxy sequencing devised by Sanger and colleagues. Both methods require amplification of target DNA either by cloning or by PCR.

An outline of dideoxy sequencing is shown in Fig. 3.22. The template is single-stranded DNA to which has been annealed a short oligonucleotide primer complementary to the region adjacent to the sequence to be determined. The primer acts as a starting point for a DNA polymerase – either a proteolytically derived fragment of DNA polymerase (Klenow fragment) or a chemically modified bacteriophage enzyme known as Sequenase* – which catalyses the sequential addition of the appropriate nucleotide to the growing chain. The reaction is carried out simultaneously in four tubes, in each of which there is a mixture of nucleotides, one of which is radiolabelled. The key aspect of the sequencing reaction is to stop chain extension at different chain lengths by adding a different dideoxynucleotide to each tube. The dideoxy triphosphates of adenine, guanine, cytosine and thymine (ddA, ddG, ddC, ddT) are incorporated into the growing chain in place of the normal nucleotides and arrest enzymatic synthesis because they lack a 3'-hydroxyl group necessary for further extension.

By mixing dideoxy and normal nucleotides in each tube at an appropriate ratio, it is possible to generate a series of fragments whose lengths indicate the position of the normal nucleotides in the DNA sequence. The four sets of reactions are then electrophoresed in adjacent slots on a long acrylamide gel and the sequence of the DNA deduced from the positions of the autoradiographic bands (Fig. 3.22).

ANALYSIS OF RNA

The techniques described in preceding sections have been concerned with the analysis of DNA, the material in which mutations occur and in which normal and genetic variation is transmitted through the generations. Much of this variation occurs in DNA whose function is not known, and which is not transcribed into RNA or translated into protein. However, genes that have metabolic function are both trans-

---

* Sequenase is a registered Trade Mark of United States Biochemicals, U.S. Patent No. 4,795,699.

cribed and translated, and a complete description of their mutations may require analysis of the corresponding mRNA and the ways in which mRNA structure and function is disturbed. Many aspects of RNA analysis are very similar to those of DNA analysis, but there are special features that need more detailed examination.

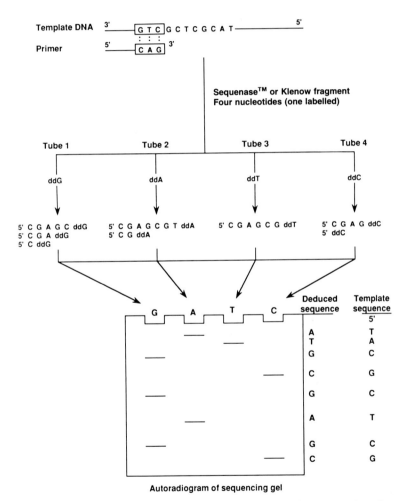

Autoradiogram of sequencing gel

Fig. 3.22. Dideoxy sequencing of DNA. The primer is annealed to the template DNA immediately adjacent to the sequence to be determined. Note that the sequence deduced from the positions of bands on the gel shows the complementary strand structure.

Northern blotting

In northern blotting or transfer, mRNA is the target material for hybridization. A very similar sequence of manipulations is used as in Southern blotting (see Fig. 3.13). The main differences are:

1 Fragmentation of RNA is usually unnecessary, since mRNA species are in the size range appropriate for electrophoresis and transfer.
2 Prior denaturation is necessary to disrupt the secondary structure that is unique to each mRNA species and which would otherwise interfere with electrophoretic separation. Electrophoresis is also carried out under denaturing conditions.

The resulting filter is then hybridized to an appropriate labelled DNA probe. The size of the RNA can be estimated by correlating the band positions with marker RNA fragments of known molecular weight. An estimate of the amount of RNA in the sample can be gauged from the intensity of the autoradiographic signal. A particular mRNA species can also be estimated directly without electrophoresis by using dot or slot blot hybridization.

Nuclease S_1 protection assays

Northern blotting gives information on the approximate size of an mRNA transcript but does not indicate the 5' or 3' ends with precision or provide data on the exon–intron structure of the DNA from which the mRNA transcript is derived. Exact definition of some mutations requires a more searching analysis than that provided by the techniques already described. One way of doing this is by forming hybrids between mRNA and a complementary DNA probe of known structure, and then using nucleases that specifically degrade single-stranded DNA or RNA but which leave double-stranded structures intact. Nuclease S_1 from *Aspergillus oryzae* is a favoured enzyme. The extent to which the RNA protects the radiolabelled DNA probe from degradation indicates the structure of the RNA. A simplified procedure for mapping the 5' terminus (or cap) of a specific mRNA transcript is shown in Fig. 3.23.

Nuclease-protection assays can also be used to map the exon structure of a transcribed gene. Processed mRNA, from which the exons have been removed, is hybridized to genomic DNA (Fig. 3.24). The hybrid molecules contains loops of intron DNA, which can be degraded by nuclease S_1. If the mixture is electrophoresed on a

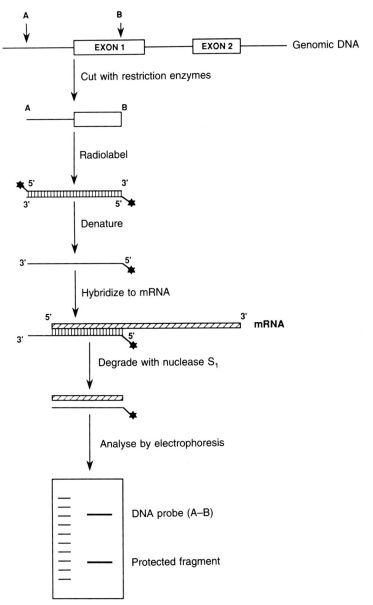

Fig. 3.23. Use of the nuclease-protection assay to map the 5′ terminus (or cap) of an mRNA. The starting material is genomic DNA from which the transcript is derived. The exact site of cleavage by restriction enzyme B must be known. The cleaved DNA is radiolabelled, denatured and hybridized to the mRNA. Nuclease S_1 digests the single-stranded regions of both DNA and RNA. The size of the protected fragment, estimated from markers on the gel, gives the distance of the 5′ terminus of the mRNA from restriction site B.

65

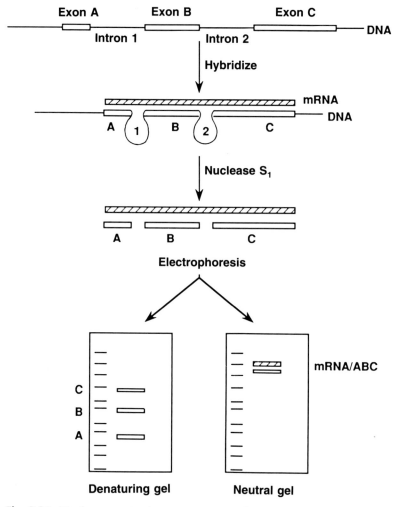

Fig. 3.24. Nuclease-protection assay to map the exon structure of a gene. Processed mRNA hybridizes to only the exons of the DNA, leaving looped introns, which are susceptible to digestion by nuclease S_1. The approximate size and number of exons can be deduced from comparison with apparent molecular weight markers on the denaturing gel, after blotting and hybridization to a radiolabelled probe.

denaturing gel and hybridized to a labelled cDNA or genomic probe from the same gene, the resulting bands will show the approximate size of the original exons. On a non-denaturing gel the hybrid will migrate as a single band indicating the size of the mRNA transcript.

Nuclease-protection assays may also be used to map exon–intron boundaries and the 3′ termini of mRNAs. These assays are not without artefacts, and may need to be backed up by more sophisticated techniques such as primer extension or run-on transcription, details of which can be found in specialist textbooks.

CLONING GENES

It was pointed out earlier in this chapter that both genomic and cDNA probes may be amplified in the laboratory by cloning into a suitable vector (such as a plasmid) that will then replicate autonomously in a host bacterial cell. The objective is to obtain multiple, identical copies of the probe, which may then be tagged and used as analytical reagents. This aspect of cloning ignores the interesting question of where the original DNA sequences come from, and how it is known that they represent genes, parts of genes or anonymous segments. In other words, how does one set about cloning a gene of interest without a friendly collaborator to provide the initial probe?

The science of gene cloning is quite complex, and only a superficial account is given here of some of the procedures in use. A key step is usually the initial preparation of libraries or clone banks in which fragmented DNA is inserted into an appropriate vector for replication in a host bacterial cell. This is similar to the scheme outlined in Fig. 3.9, except that each colony may now contain a different recombinant DNA sequence. The objective in creating a library is to have all the original inserted DNA sequences represented at least once in the final collection of colonies. In practice this is difficult to achieve, and several different libraries may need to be prepared to increase the chances of total representation. However, once created, libraries are permanent resources and may be used repeatedly in further experiments.

There are two main types of library, prepared from either genomic DNA or cDNA. Genomic libraries are made by fractionating all the DNA from a suitable cell and this, in principle, can represent the entire human genome. To handle such large amounts of DNA, digestion is often carried out with rare-cutter restriction enzymes (which cleave at infrequent recognition sites) and the large fragments incorporated into specialized vectors such as cosmids or yeast artificial chromosomes (YACs). YAC libraries, in which the host cell is the yeast *Saccharomyces cerevisiae,* have been created with an average insert size of 350 kb, a huge increase on the maximum 10 kb insert of a plasmid vector. If the size of the human haploid genome is taken as 3×10^9 bp and the average insert size as 350 000 bp (350 kb), the entire genome could in theory be represented in as few as 8000 recombinant clones. In practice, about three to five times this number of clones is

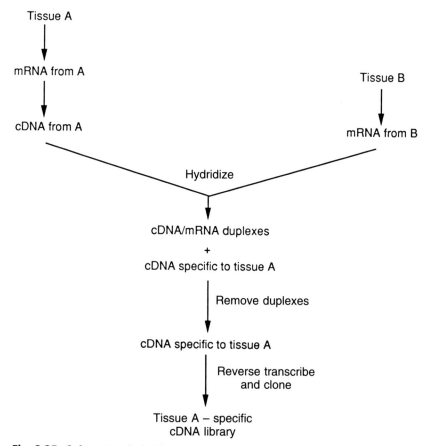

Fig. 3.25. Subtractive hybridization to enrich for cDNA for a particular tissue. mRNA from tissue A is reverse transcribed into single-stranded cDNA, which is then hybridized to mRNA from tissue B. Duplex cDNA–mRNA is removed using hydroxylapatite, and the remaining cDNA, largely specific to tissue A, reverse transcribed into double-stranded cDNA and cloned into a suitable vector.

needed to increase the chance of finding a particular unique fragment. Genomic libraries can be simplified by initially fractionating chromosomes on a fluorescence-activated cell sorter, and selecting only one chromosome for digestion and insertion.

cDNA libraries differ from genomic libraries in that they are based on the mRNA of a particular tissue. To prepare a liver cDNA library, for example, the mRNA of liver is reverse transcribed into cDNA (Fig. 3.10), and then double-stranded cDNA fragmented and inserted into an appropriate vector. However, most tissues contain many mRNA species in common, and such a liver cDNA library would not be particularly liver-specific, although it might be enriched in cDNAs representing the more abundant liver mRNAs. Specificity can be increased by an initial subtractive hybridization procedure (Fig. 3.25), in which mRNA from another cell type is used to remove sequences that are common to the two tissues. It is also possible to enrich for particular mRNA sequences, using a tissue in which they are abundantly expressed, by precipitating polysomes with specific antibodies, before the creation of a cDNA library.

Once the library has been prepared, the next step is to isolate the recombinant clone representing the gene of interest. This is much easier to achieve if something is known about the encoded protein product. In general, only a partial amino acid sequence is required and this can be deduced by microsequencing of very small quantities of purified protein. Knowledge of the genetic code (Table 3.2) will allow construction of a set of oligonucleotides that match the predicted sequence coding for the particular region of the protein. (Because of degeneracy in the code, a set of oligonucleotides rather than a single oligonucleotide is necessary.) The oligonucleotide set is radio-labelled and then hybridized to the library (preferably a cDNA library prepared from a tissue in which the protein is abundant), which has been spread out as colonies on a plate. Clones giving a positive hybridization signal are picked out and grown up. With luck, skill and some repetition, such clones will contain at least part of the gene of interest. Sequencing (Fig. 3.22) will confirm whether or not this is the case.

It is more difficult, but not impossible, to clone genes whose protein products are unknown, and whose existence is often inferred solely through a disease phenotype. A classical example is the cystic fibrosis gene, whose encoded protein product defied analysis over a 40-year period of quite intense investigation. Such genes can be cloned only by reverse genetics or positional cloning. The first step is to establish genetic linkage to DNA markers (Chapter 5) and then to

REVERSE GENETICS
(positional cloning)

Mendelian disorder with clear mode of inheritance

↓

Search for DNA markers cosegregating with disease locus

↓

Establish firm genetic linkage to a marker

↓

Use DNA marker to localize disease gene locus to a specific region
of a chromosome

↓

Continue search for more closely linked markers

↓

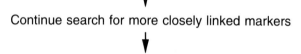

Chromosome jumping and walking to move towards disease gene
locus

↓

Clone gene and determine nucleotide sequence

↓

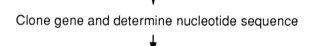

Compare nucleotide sequences in DNA from normal and affected
individuals

↓

Infer amino acid sequence of protein product of normal and disease
genes

↓

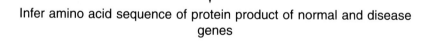

Isolate protein product of normal and disease genes

Fig. 3.26. A schematic outline of reverse genetics or positional cloning. See
the text for details.

map the whole group to a specific chromosomal region (Chapter 7). A search is then continued for more closely linked DNA markers, ideally bracketing the disease gene locus, and perhaps even showing a phenomenon known as linkage disequilibrium (Chapter 5). Close markers provide a starting point for fairly sophisticated new manipulations known as chromosome walking and jumping, in which successive sequences between the markers are examined for evidence of functional genes. Once a candidate gene is identified, it can be cloned and sequenced, and the function of the encoded product deduced by analysis of homologies with other known genes. This may lead to rejection of the candidate gene as being of the wrong type, and thus to a continued search for further candidates. The final step is a demonstration that the isolated gene has a systematic difference in sequence (perhaps only a single nucleotide change) between affected and unaffected individuals. An outline of reverse genetic cloning is shown in Fig. 3.26.

SUGGESTED READING

Berger, S. L. and Kimmel A. R. (Editors) (1987). *Guide to molecular cloning techniques. Methods in Enzymology*, Vol. 152, Academic Press, San Diego, CA.

Bishop, M. J. and Rawlings, C. J. (Editors) (1987). *Nucleic Acid and Protein Sequence Analysis: a Practical Approach*. IRL Press, Oxford.

Davies, K. E. (Editor) (1986). *Human Genetic Diseases: a Practical Approach*. IRL Press, Oxford.

Davies, K. E. (Editor) (1988). *Genome Analysis: a Practical Approach*. IRL Press, Oxford.

Davies, K. E. and Read, A. P. (1988). *Molecular Basis of Inherited Disease*. IRL Press, Oxford.

Erlich, H. A., Gibbs, R. and Kazazian, H. H. (Editors) (1989). *Polymerase Chain Reaction*. Cold Spring Harbor Laboratory Press, Cold Spring Harbor, NY.

Innis, M. A., Gelfand, D. H., Sninsky, J. J. and Wight, T. J. (Editors) (1990). *PCR Protocols: a Guide to Methods and Applications*. Academic Press, San Diego, CA.

Kingsman, S. M. and Kingsman, A. J. (1988). *Genetic Engineering*. Blackwell Scientific Publications, Oxford.

Lewin, B. (1990). *Genes IV*. Oxford University Press, Oxford.

Old, R. W. and Primrose, S. B. (1989). *Principles of Gene Manipulation*. 4th Edition, Blackwell Scientific Publications, Oxford.

Sambrook, J., Fritsch, E. F. and Maniatis, T. (1989). *Molecular Cloning: a Laboratory Manual*. 2nd Edition, Cold Spring Harbor Laboratory Press, Cold Spring Harbor, NY.

Singer, M. and Berg, P. (1991). *Genes and Genomes: a Changing Perspective*. Blackwell Scientific Publications, Oxford.

4 MUTATION

MUTATIONS AND GENETIC VARIATION

In a broad sense, a mutation is any change involving the genetic material, DNA. There are three major categories of mutation (Table 4.1). Genome mutations affect the number of chromosomes in the cell. In polyploidy there is the addition of one or more haploid sets of 23 chromosomes, whereas in aneuploidy there is gain or loss of individual chromosomes. In chromosome mutations there are microscopically visible alterations in the structure of chromosomes, in the form of deletions, duplications, inversions and translocations. These two categories of mutation belong to the discipline of cyto-genetics and are discussed in Chapter 7. In this chapter, I concentrate on gene mutations, the subtle or not-so-subtle alterations that occur in discrete sequences of coding or non-coding DNA.

The mutations giving rise to genetic diseases are usually inherited and pass unchanged from one generation to the next. It is one of the axioms of molecular genetics that a particular defined mutation is likely to be the same in all members of an immediate family. None the less, mutations can arise de novo in the germ cells of the parent and appear without warning in an affected child. Such new mutations are frequently found in X-linked recessive conditions and in severe con-ditions with autosomal dominant inheritance. If the affected individual reproduces, the new mutation will now be inherited according to the rules of Mendelian transmission.

Occasionally mutations arise in the differentiated tissues rather than in the germ cells. Such somatic mutations are not inherited. They are of particular importance in the origins of tumours and are discussed in Chapter 6.

Mutations are usually regarded as harmful, and in general this is true. Highly evolved and complex organisms, such as humans, can tolerate only limited change to their genetic material without dis-astrous consequences. All genome mutations and a majority of chromosome mutations, though potentially heritable, are in fact

73

Table 4.1. *Major categories of mutation*

Genome mutations	Alteration in the number of chromosomes; polyploidy involves whole diploid sets; aneuploidy involves gain or loss of individual chromosomes
Chromosome mutations	Microscopically visible alterations in the structure of chromosomes, i.e. deletions, duplications, inversions, translocations
Gene mutations	More subtle changes in the structure of a coding gene or non-coding DNA sequence

genetic lethals and are usually seen as de novo events. None the less, human populations are very heterogeneous in their genetic make-up, and the types of mutation giving rise to such normal variation must have been either selectively neutral or beneficial in the appropriate environment.

It has been apparent for many years that some genes can have alternative forms (alleles), no one of which is more normal than any other. The existence of alternative alleles at a single genetic locus is known as genetic polymorphism. The first such polymorphism to be clearly defined in humans was the ABO blood group system, described as early as 1900. In subsequent years, an extensive panoply of polymorphisms was discovered and catalogued. However, the advent of molecular genetic techniques has vastly increased our understanding of both the extent and the nature of genetic variation in human populations. It has become possible to search the human genome for variation in those regions of DNA that are neither transcribed nor expressed in protein. The range of this type of silent variation continues to unfold, and has been quite unexpected in its extent and complexity. Its existence constitutes an extremely powerful tool both for unravelling the structure of the human genome and for tracking expressed genes responsible for pathological variation.

In this chapter, mutation is considered in two sections. I first discuss the types of mutation responsible for single-gene defects, drawing examples for some of the better-known Mendelian disorders. Because of their historical importance in illuminating the molecular pathology of mutation, the haemoglobinopathies provide many of the best-studied examples. In the second section, I review the subject of DNA polymorphism, the types of silent mutation that continue to provide molecular genetics with one of its most powerful working tools.

MUTATIONS AND PATHOLOGICAL VARIATION
GENE DELETIONS

α-Thalassaemia was referred to briefly in Chapter 3 (Fig. 3.15). There are two clinically important forms of this disorder; Hb H disease, in which individuals have moderate to severe anaemia and produce an unusual haemoglobin (Hb H) consisting of β-globin tetramers (β_4), and hydrops fetalis, which leads to stillbirth or neonatal death and in which the fetus has a haemoglobin (Hb Barts) consisting of γ-globin tetramers (γ_4). In Hb H disease, there is reduced production of α-globin chains, and the imbalance in synthesis of α- and β-globin chains results in an excess of β-chains and the unusual β_4 molecule. In hydrops fetalis, there is complete absence of α-globin synthesis, so that the fetus cannot make haemoglobin F ($\alpha_2\gamma_2$) and instead produces the γ_4 molecule of Hb Barts, which has virtually no oxygen-carrying capacity.

Interpretation of these findings came from the discovery that there are two α-globin genes in the human genome, situated contiguously on each chromosome 16. Hb H disease arises when only one of the four α-globin genes is functional, and hydrops fetalis when there are no functional α-globin genes (Fig. 4.1). There are three possible heterozygous states; in one, a single α-globin gene is non-functional and such individuals are referred to as silent carriers. The other heterozygous states differ in whether the two non-functional α-globin genes are present on a single chromosome ($\alpha\alpha/--$) or on different chromosomes ($\alpha-/\alpha-$). If both parents are $\alpha\alpha/--$ heterozygotes, they have a one in four chance of a child with hydrops fetalis ($--/--$). If one parent is $\alpha\alpha/--$ and the other $\alpha-/\alpha-$, there is a one in four risk of Hb H disease. One would expect both Hb H and hydrops fetalis in siblings only if one parent were $\alpha\alpha/--$ and the other parent had Hb H disease ($\alpha-/--$).

Molecular studies have shown that most cases of α-thalassaemia are due to gene deletions. The extent of the different deletions is variable and involves a number of segments of the α-globin cluster on chromosome 16 (Fig. 4.2). Deletion of a single α-gene or parts of both α-genes (which leaves a composite residual α-gene) permits some α-globin synthesis and an α^+ phenotype. More extensive deletions, some of which remove the pseudo-alpha (ψα), pseudo-zeta (ψζ) or zeta (ζ) genes upstream, destroy globin synthesis and lead to α⁰ phenotypes. The ζ-gene product is a constituent of the embryonic haemoglobins, Gower 1 and Portland.

The deletion of a single α-globin gene arises from unequal crossing-over between homologous chromosomes 16 during meiosis. If the two chromosomes misalign so that the α1-gene on one is paired with the α2 on the other (Fig. 4.3), the outcome is a chromosome with one

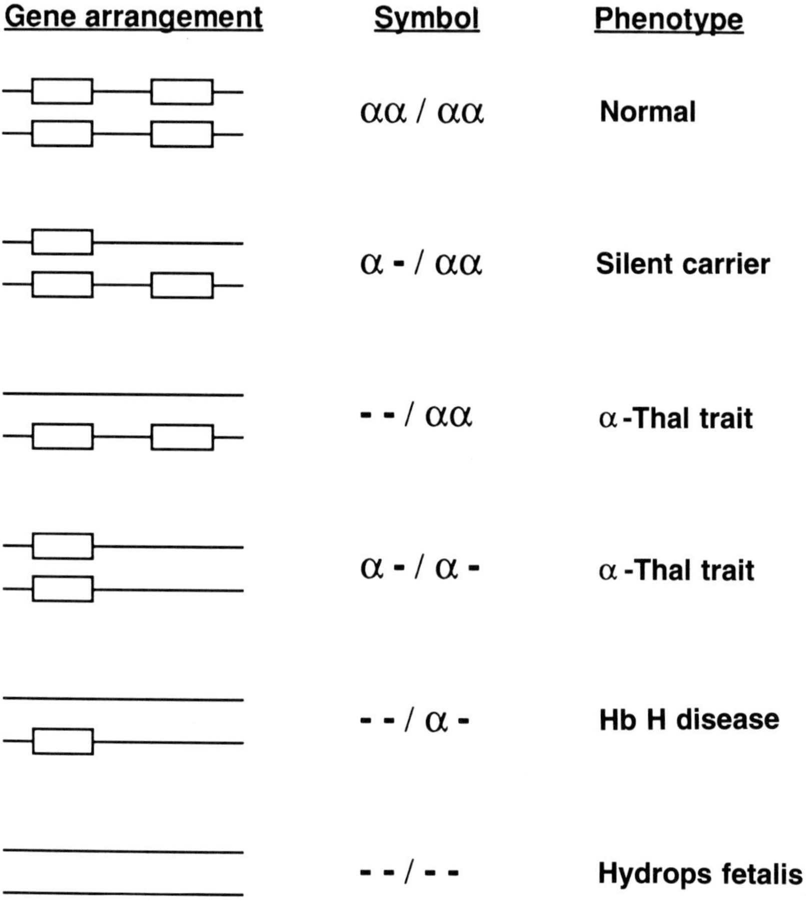

Gene arrangement	Symbol	Phenotype
	αα / αα	Normal
	α - / αα	Silent carrier
	- - / αα	α -Thal trait
	α - / α -	α -Thal trait
	- - / α -	Hb H disease
	- - / - -	Hydrops fetalis

Fig. 4.1. The genetic basis of α-thalassamia (α-thal). The normal α-globin genes are shown as open boxes and deleted genes as single lines. There are three different heterozygous states; silent carrier and the two different types of α-thal trait.

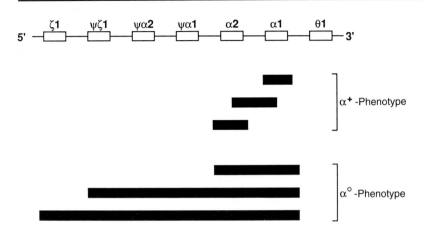

Fig. 4.2. Schematic representation of the α-globin gene cluster on chromosome 16 (top), and illustrative examples of gene deletions (filled bars) leading to α^+ or α^0 phenotypes. Not drawn to scale.

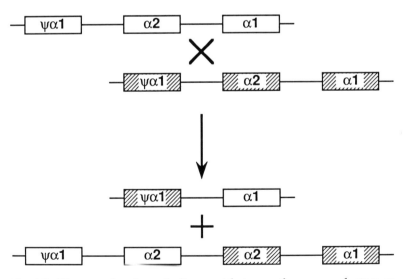

Fig. 4.3. Diagram showing misalignment between the α-gene clusters on homologous chromosomes, followed by unequal crossing-over. One chromosome now has a single functional α-globin gene (α1), while the other has three functional α-globin genes (α2, α2, α1).

α-gene and a chromosome with three α-genes. The triple α-gene chromosome has been found in many different populations, and some homozygous individuals with six α-globin genes have been encountered. Molecular explanations for the loss of both α-genes from a chromosome cannot easily be devised on the unequal crossing-over model.

Major deletions in the β-globin cluster give rise to two related conditions, hereditary persistence of fetal haemoglobin (HPFH) and δβ-thalassaemia. Several different forms of HPFH are known, characterized by a deletion of both δ- and β-genes that extends some distance to the 3' end of the cluster (Fig. 4.4). In such individuals the γ-globin gene, instead of switching off in early postnatal life, continues to produce γ-globin chains throughout adulthood and thus Hb F ($α_2γ_2$) compensates for the absent δ- and β-globin synthesis. In contrast, in the δβ-thalassaemias, some of which involve quite similar gene deletions within the cluster, there is insufficient compensatory γ-globin synthesis to overcome the absence of δ- and β-globin chains, and the clinical consequence is a moderate to severe thalassaemia. Why some deletions in this cluster lead to the benign HPFH and others to a quite severe thalassaemia is not understood.

PARTIAL GENE DELETIONS
The deletion of a complete gene obviously precludes the possibility of any production of its protein product. Partial gene deletions,

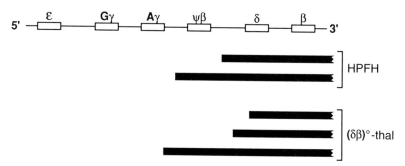

Fig. 4.4. Schematic representation of the β-globin gene cluster on chromosome 11 (top), together with examples of deletions (solid bars; broken edges indicate the extent of the deletions lie further in a 3' direction) leading to hereditary persistence of fetal haemoglobin (HPFH) or δβ-thalassaemias. For reasons that are not yet clear, very similar deletions can lead to the benign HPFH or a severe thalassaemia.

however, still allow for some protein synthesis, even if the resulting protein is truncated or grossly altered. Illustrative examples of partial gene deletions and their biochemical consequences have emerged recently from studies of the mutations responsible for the X-linked muscular dystrophies.

The cloning of the muscular dystrophy gene in 1987 confirmed earlier evidence from linkage analysis that the two clinically distinct conditions, Duchenne muscular dystrophy (DMD) and Becker muscular dystrophy (BMD), are caused by mutations in the same dystrophin gene. This is the largest gene yet identified in humans and spans more than 2500 kb of genomic DNA (almost 1% of the X chromosome), comprising more than 70 exons. The enormous size of the gene goes some way towards explaining the high mutation rate in these disorders, with up to one-third of the cases representing new mutations.

Molecular analysis has demonstrated that a majority of cases of both DMD and BMD are caused by partial deletions of the dystrophin gene. There appear to be at least two preferential deletion hotspots, one to the 5' end of the gene between exons 6 and 7, and the other located more centrally, between exons 44 and 45 (Fig. 4.5). Little correlation has been found between the extent of the deletion and clinical severity; some mild cases of BMD who were still ambulant at advanced age were shown to have large portions of their dystrophin gene deleted, while some severe cases of DMD who were chair-bound by age 13 had relatively minor deletions. Very similar proportions of deletions (50% to 70%) were found amongst the mutations responsible for the two conditions.

In order to explain the considerable variation in clinical severity between DMD and BMD, it has been suggested that a key factor is whether the genomic deletion alters the reading frame of the resulting mRNA. As indicated earlier, the genetic code is read in triplets of nucleotide bases (codons), so that a break that occurs within a codon can create a completely new reading frame to the 3' end of the mRNA, that is the subsequent sequence is read out of frame. In contrast, a break that removes a complete codon or group of complete codons will lead to an interruption of amino acid sequence, but is then followed by the expected sequence of amino acid residues. An illustration of this phenomenon is shown in Fig. 4.6. There is now good evidence that most of the differences between DMD and BMD can be explained in this way, with a majority of severe DMD deletions interrupting the reading frame, whereas most BMD deletions leave it intact. The use of specific antibodies to detect dystrophin molecules

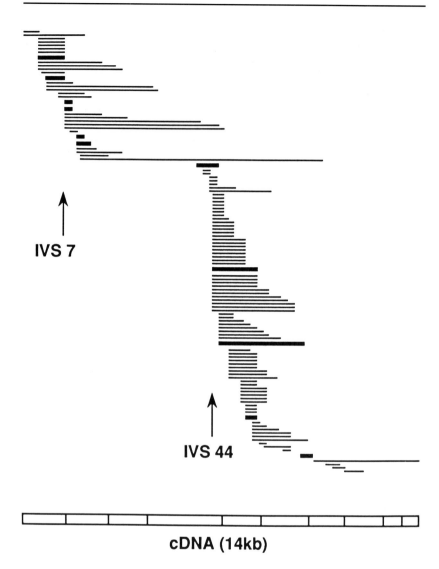

cDNA (14kb)

Fig. 4.5. A schematic representation of partial deletions and duplications of the dystrophin gene leading to DMD and BMD. Mutation hotspots are found in intron 7 (IVS7) and intron 44 (IVS44). The 14 kb cDNA, divided into segments commonly used as individual probes, is shown below for reference and allows a rough estimate of the extent of deleted coding material.

in muscle tissue confirms this hypothesis, with most BMD patients having measurable levels of semi-functional protein and most DMD having no detectable dystrophin.

CODON DELETIONS

Small deletions that remove an entire codon or a small set of entire codons will not alter the reading frame of the mRNA, but will lead to a protein product from which one or more amino acid residues will be absent. Several variant haemoglobin molecules are known where this

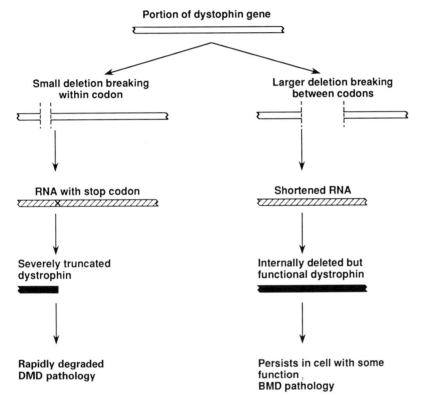

Fig. 4.6. Diagram indicating how disruption of the reading frame explains differences in the pathology of DMD and BMD. Deletions breaking within codons, even when comparatively small, may generate a stop codon (X) in the transcribed RNA and encode a severely truncated dystrophin protein that is rapidly degraded by the cell. Deletions that do not interrupt the reading frame may lead to internally deleted, but still functional, dystrophin protein with consequent milder pathology.

has happened; most involve the β-globin rather than the α-globin gene. The resulting haemoglobin is characterized by instability or altered affinity for oxygen, and in the heterozygous state may lead to mild haemolytic anaemia or erythrocytosis. Of particular interest is the abnormal haemoglobin known as Gun Hill, which lacks five amino acid residues at positions 91–95 in the β-chain. A plausible explanation suggests misalignment during meiosis of codons 91–94 in one chromosome with the closely matched codons 96–98 in the homologous chromosome (Fig. 4.7). After recombination, this would lead to a clean deletion of five codons on one chromosome (Gun Hill), and a theoretical possibility of the duplication of five codons on the other. Although no variant haemoglobin has been discovered with exactly this five codon duplication, other haemoglobins are known with small duplications that could have arisen by a similar mechanism.

One recently discovered small deletion is responsible for a majority of cases of the recessively inherited disorder cystic fibrosis (CF). The

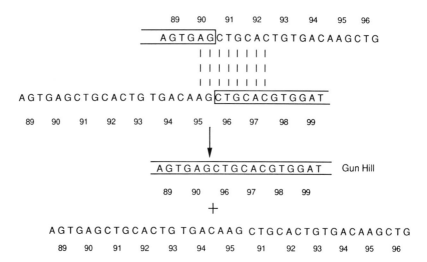

Fig. 4.7. Derivation of haemoglobin Gun Hill by mispairing of homologous chromosomes during meiosis and subsequent unequal crossing-over. Note the similarities between codons 91 to 94 and 96 to 99, the presumed origin of the mispairing. In the resulting gene for Hb Gun Hill, codons 91 to 95 are deleted. There is also a theoretical possibility of an abnormal haemoglobin in which codons 91 to 95 would be duplicated.

deletion of three nucleotides, CTT in exon 10 of the CF gene,* is strictly speaking out of frame, since it affects parts of two adjacent codons (Fig. 4.8). However, because of degeneracy of the genetic code, the new fusion codon ATT continues to specify isoleucine, and the net consequence of the deletion is the removal of a single amino acid residue, phenylalanine, at position 508 in the 1480 amino acid residues that comprise the protein product of the CF gene. This deletion, called ΔF_{508}, occurs in 50% to 80% of CF chromosomes, depending on the population surveyed, and is easily detectable on an electrophoresis gel after amplification of part of exon 10 (see Fig. 3.19).

DUPLICATIONS AND INSERTIONS

It has been pointed out that unequal crossing-over during meiosis is a probable mechanism for the deletion of whole genes or parts of genes (Figs. 4.3 and 4.7). This process can also generate duplications, as in the classical example of the triplicate α-globin genes found in some populations. Partial gene duplications have also been described amongst the mutations responsible for DMD and BMD and may

Codon no.	505	506	507	508	509	510
Normal codons	AAT	ATC	ATC	TTT	GGT	GTT
Normal amino acids	asn	ile	ile	phe	gly	val
ΔF_{508} codons	AAT	ATC	AT-	---	TGG	TGTT
ΔF_{508} amino acids	asn	ile		ile	gly	val

Fig. 4.8. A codon deletion in exon 10 of the CF gene that is responsible for a majority of cases of this disorder. The deletion removes the third base of codon 507 and the first two bases of codon 508. The new composite codon ATT continues to specify isoleucine, so that the net effect is the removal of a single amino acid residue, phenylalanine, at position 508.

* More exactly, this gene codes for a protein known as the cystic fibrosis transmembrane conductance regulator (CFTR). Since it has been defined by mutations giving rise to CF, it is conveniently called the CF gene. The exact function of CFTR is yet to be established.

83

represent up to 5% of all cases. The clinical consequence of such duplications depends on whether the insertion of additional sequences disrupts the codon reading frame of the mutant gene.

FUSION MUTATIONS

Unequal crossing-over between non-homologous genes can also result in a class of fusion gene mutations. These are best illustrated by defects in colour vision genes leading to different kinds of colour blindness. Humans have three different colour genes; a blue pigment gene on chromosome 7 and contiguous red and green pigment genes at the tip of the long arm of the X chromosome. There is a single red pigment gene but one to three (occasionally more) green pigment genes situated to the 3' side of the red gene. Red and green pigment genes are highly homologous and are assumed to have evolved from a common ancestral red pigment gene.

X-linked colour-vision defects affect about 8% of Caucasian males, with deuteranopia (green-colour blindedness) being some three times as common as protanopia (red-colour blindedness). Many different types of mutation account for these defects, but among the more interesting are fusion genes resulting from unequal crossing-over between red and green pigment genes. In the example shown in Fig. 4.9, meiotic misalignment of a red pigment gene on one X chromo-

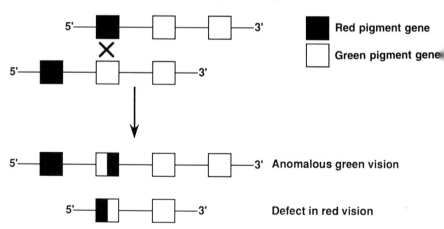

Fig. 4.9. Schematic representation of meiotic misalignment and unequal crossing-over between X-linked red and green colour-vision genes. Two fusion genes result, in one case resulting in anomalous green vision (the chromosome still has two normal green pigment genes) and in the other defective red vision (no intact red pigment gene).

some with a green pigment gene on another will produce two fusion genes, one associated with deficient red vision and the other with anomalous green vision in males inheriting these chromosomes.

POINT MUTATIONS

In molecular terms, the simplest type of mutation is a base substitution, the replacement of one base-pair in double-stranded DNA by a different base-pair. If the mutation involves the substitution of one pyrimidine by another (e.g. C→T) or one purine by another (e.g. A→G) it is called a transition. When a purine is replaced by a pyrimidine, or vice versa, it is known as a transversion. Transitions are more common than transversions. Such point mutations naturally involve both DNA strands, so that a C→T transition in the sense strand would be followed by a G→A change in the antisense strand. There is evidence for mutational hotspots in the human genome with the dinucleotide CG (also written CpG to indicate polarity) being particularly prone to point mutations.

Because of the degeneracy of the genetic code, not all base substitutions lead to an alteration in the amino acid residue specified. Often the third base in the codon is not significant (see Table 3.1), and third base degeneracy minimizes the effect of mutations. Silent substitutions leading to synonymous codons probably account for up to one-third of all point mutations.

Missense mutations

A base substitution that alters the amino acid residue coded for by the particular three-base codon is called a missense mutation. Not all missense mutations have pathological consequences and base substitutions that generate codons specifying a new amino acid residue with properties similar to those of the replaced residue may have little effect on the properties of the protein. The base substitution CUU→AUU leads to a change from one neutral hydrophobic residue leucine to another neutral hydrophobic residue isoleucine, and GAU→GAA replaces the acidic residue aspartic acid with the acidic residue glutamic acid (see Table 3.1).

The first missense mutation to be defined in a human gene that results in pathological consequences was the single-base substitution in codon six of the β-globin gene leading to sickle cell anaemia (Fig. 4.10). GAG in the sense strand of the DNA codes for the acidic residue glutamic acid. A transversion from A to T in the second base of the codon results in a codon change to GTG, which specifies (via the mRNA codon GUG) the neutral and hydrophobic residue valine.

Thus normal haemoglobin A and haemoglobin S differ by a single amino acid at position 6 in the β-globin chain, the direct result of a single base-pair change. All the devastating consequences of sickle cell anaemia may be traced to this small alteration. Another relatively common abnormal haemoglobin, Hb C, results from a transition in codon six of the β-globin gene, in this case GAG→AAG and glutamic acid to lysine (Fig. 4.10).

A large number of missense mutations have been described in the haemoglobin molecule, affecting both α- and β-globin chains. In general, the resulting pathology is not as severe as that associated with more drastic changes in gene structure (there are some notable exceptions to this broad statement, e.g. sickle cell anaemia). Likewise, missense mutations in other genes may also result in comparatively mild disease. One example is α_1-antitrypsin deficiency, a relatively common recessively inherited condition amongst Caucasians, which may lead to childhood liver cirrhosis or early-onset emphysema. A missense mutation in exon V of the gene (GAG→AAG) results in a glutamic acid to lysine substitution at position 342 of the α_1-antitrypsin protein (Fig. 4.11). The resulting Z protein is processed and secreted poorly by the liver and is not as effective as the normal M protein in inhibiting neutrophil elastase.

Codon no.	5	6	7
β^A-Gene	CCT	GAG	GAG
β^A-Globin	pro	glu	glu
β^S-Gene	CCT	GⲮG	GAG
β^S-Globin	pro	val	glu
β^C-Gene	CCT	ⲮAG	GAG
β^C-Globin	pro	lys	glu

Fig. 4.10. Two missense mutations at codon 6 of the β-globin gene. The normal codon (β^A gene) is GAG, specifying glutamic acid. A transversion GAG→GTG in the β^S gene leads to replacement of glutamic acid by valine. A transition GAG→AAG in the β^C gene leads to replacement of glutamic acid by lysine.

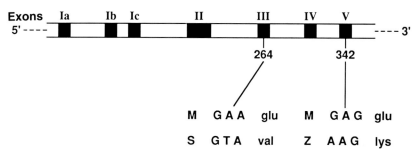

Fig. 4.11. Missense mutations in the α_1-antitrypsin gene. In codon 264 in exon III there is a GAA→GTA change, which substitutes glutamic acid in the normal M protein with valine in the S protein. In codon 342 in exon V a GAG→AAG change replaces glutamic acid in the normal M protein with lysine in the Z protein.

None the less, a majority of ZZ homozygotes live relatively normal lives and may delay the onset of emphysema by resolute avoidance of cigarette smoking. The other common mutation in the α_1-antitrypsin gene is also a missense change, with a GAA to GTA transversion in exon III, leading to a glutamic acid to valine substitution at position 264. The resulting S protein is a relatively benign variant, except when found with the Z protein in SZ compound heterozygotes.

Nonsense mutations
A potentially disruptive point mutation is one that converts an amino acid-specifying codon to a stop codon. If the mutation occurs near the 5' end of the gene, the resulting polypeptide will be severely truncated and be without function or rapidly degraded by the cell. One of the more common mutations leading to β-thalassaemia amongst Mediterranean populations is such a nonsense mutation in the second exon of the β-globin gene. This is a C→T transition in the first base of codon 39 and produces a stop codon in place of a glutamic acid residue (Fig. 4.12). The consequence of this mutation is the absence of any recognizable β-globin chains.

Several nonsense mutations have also been described in the factor VIII gene responsible for haemophilia A. The factor VIII gene is large and spans 186 kb with 26 exons and 25 introns. About 10% of patients with haemophilia A develop antibodies against exogenous factor VIII used in replacement therapy; this is thought to arise when the patients have no endogenous factor VIII and their immune systems see the infused material as a foreign protein. In most haemophilia A

87

Codon no.	36	37	38	39	40	41
β^A-Gene	CCT	TGG	ACC	C̲AG	AGG	TTC
RNA codons	CCU	UGG	ACC	CAG	AGG	UUC
β^A-Globin	pro	trp	thr	glu	arg	phe
β°_{39}-Gene	CCT	TGG	ACC	T̲AG	AGG	TTC
RNA Codons	CCU	UGG	ACC	UAG	AGG	UUC
β°_{39}-Globin	pro	trp	thr	STOP		

Fig. 4.12. A nonsense mutation in codon 39 of the β-globin gene. The C→T transition (underlined) creates a new codon TAG, which signals (through the RNA codon UAG) termination of translation. The truncated β-globin is not recognizable in the cell and the consequence is a β^0-thalassaemia phenotype.

patients where the defect in the factor VIII gene is due to nonsense mutations such antibodies have been found, even though the nonsense mutation occurs in exons towards the 3′ end of the gene. One striking example of the destructive effect of a nonsense mutation has been reported in a patient with severe haemophilia A, where a C→T substitution in exon 26 removes only the carboxyl-terminal 26 amino acid residues of the 2351 amino acid residue factor VIII protein. Although no antibodies developed in this patient, it appears that the carboxyl-terminal 26 residues are crucial for ensuring the clotting activity of factor VIII.

Stop-codon mutations
The opposite of a nonsense mutation is a point substitution converting a stop codon to a codon that specifies an amino acid residue. In haemoglobin Constant Spring, the normal stop codon TAA at position 142 in the α-globin gene (UAA in mRNA) has been changed to CAA, which specifies glutamine. The consequence is that the translation machinery of the cell continues to read the mRNA until a more distal stop codon is encountered at position 173 (Fig. 4.13). Constant Spring has α-globin chains of 172 amino acid residues in place of the normal 141 residues. It is relatively unstable, produced in low quanti-

Codon no.	139 140 141 142 143 144 – – – – – 172 173

α^{A}-Codons

AA$_{G}^{A}$UACCGU$_{U}^{}$AAGCUGGA – – – – – GAAUAA

α^{A}-Globin

lys tyr arg STOP

Constant Spring codons

AA$_{G}^{A}$UACCGU$_{C}^{}$AAGCUGGA – – – – – GAAUAA

Constant Spring globin

lys tyr arg gln ala gly – – – – – glu STOP

Fig. 4.13. A point mutation in the termination codon of the α-globin gene leading to haemoglobin Constant Spring. Only RNA codons are shown. A UAA→CAA change at codon 142 alters the stop codon to one specifying glutamine. The normally untranslated region at the 3′ end of the RNA is read-through to codon 173 where another stop codon terminates translation. Three other almost identical variant haemoglobins have lysine (UAA→AAA), glutamic acid (UAA→GAA) or serine (UAA→UCA) residues at position 142 of the α-chain, but otherwise the same extra 31 amino acid residues.

ties and associated with α-thalassaemia trait. Three other, very similar, stop-codon mutations of codon 142 of the α-globin gene have been described; they are identical with Constant Spring except for the residue at position 142 of the extended α-chain.

Frameshift mutations

In the discussion of partial gene deletions responsible for DMD and BMD, reference was made to the importance of frameshifts in the structure of the residual dystrophin protein. Frameshifts can also occur as a result of point mutations, if the deletion or insertion of a single nucleotide disrupts the reading frame so that it specifies a set of new codons at the 3′ end of the gene. In most cases where the frameshift is near the 5′ end of the gene, the resulting protein will be unrecognizable and rapidly degraded. However, there are examples of frameshifts that produce novel and partially functioning proteins. One of these is haemoglobin Wayne, an α-globin variant in which a single nucleotide deletion in codon 139 enables a set of new amino acid residues at position 139 to 146 to be specified (Fig. 4.14). The α-chain of Wayne thus has an additional five amino acid residues at the carboxyl end of the protein, and terminates because of the creation of a new stop codon.

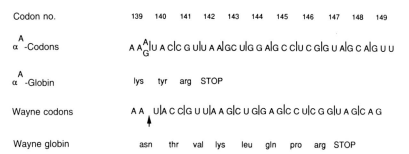

Fig. 4.14. A frameshift mutation leading to haemoglobin Wayne. Deletion of the third base in codon 139 of the α-globin gene means that the first base of the original codon 140 now becomes the third base of the new codon 139. This frameshift alters the termination codon at position 142 and there is read-through to a new termination codon at position 147. Hb Wayne thus has five extra amino acid residues and three new residues at positions 139–141.

RNA SPLICE MUTATIONS

It was pointed out in Chapter 3 that one important aspect of RNA processing is the precise splicing out of introns to produce a mature mRNA ready for translation. Nearly all eukaryotic genes have a dinucleotide GT at the 5′ starting point of the intron (the donor site) and a dinucleotide AG at the 3′ end (the acceptor site: see Fig. 3.15). Mutations in genomic DNA that alter the structure of either donor or acceptor sites in RNA interrupt normal splicing and produce a non-functional mRNA. Amongst the β-thalassaemias some 12 different splice junction mutations have been described, each of which in the homozygous state results in a phenotype with no β-globin chain production (β⁰-thalassaemia).

Further analysis of human genes has shown that there are additional nucleotide sequences at intron–exon boundaries that are important in RNA splicing. These are known as consensus sequences. At the donor site they include the last three residues in the preceding exon and the first six residues in the intron. At the acceptor site they include the last ten residues of the intron and the first residue of the following exon. The consensus sequence for the donor site of the first intron in the β-globin gene is shown in Fig. 4.15. Seven mutations affecting these nucleotides have been observed, all leading to β⁺-thalassaemia phenotypes with diminished globin production. Mutations involving the consensus sequences surrounding the acceptor sites in both the first and second β-globin gene introns also lead to β⁺-thalassaemia phenotypes.

	Exon 1	Intron 1		Exon 2	
5′	C A G $\underline{GT}$ T G G T	.... T T $\underline{AG}$ G C T	.... 3′		

Position 1	$\underline{A}$			β°
Position 1	I			β°
Position 2	$\underline{G}$			β°
Position 129		$\underline{G}$		β°
Position 5	T			β+
Position 5	C			β+
Position 5	A			β+
Position 6	C			β+
Position 128		C		β+

Fig. 4.15. Point mutations affecting splice junctions and consensus sequences of the first intron of the β-globin gene. Donor GT and acceptor AG sites are underlined. Mutations at these sites (positions 1, 2, 129 of intron 1) lead to a β°-thalassaemia phenotype. Mutations in the consensus sequences (positions 5, 6, 128) of intron 1 lead to a less severe β+-thalassaemia phenotype. Similar mutations have also been described in the second intron of the β-globin gene and in a variety of other genes.

It is also possible to find point mutations in introns, well away from the consensus regions, that create new acceptor sites for splicing. In one of the more common Mediterranean forms of β-thalassaemia there is a G→A change at position 110 of intron 1 and the creation of a new AG acceptor some 21 nucleotides to the 5′ side of the normal acceptor site (Fig. 4.16). The new acceptor site functions better than the original and is used more often than the normal site in splicing events. Since it results in a mature mRNA with an additional 19 nucleotides from intron 1, it is useless as a template for β-globin synthesis. Some normal mRNA is produced from the original acceptor site, and thus the phenotype is a β+-thalassaemia. Several other similar intron mutations have been described and are referred to as pseudosplice substitutions or internal intron changes.

There is another class of RNA-processing mutation exemplified by a South-east Asian variant haemoglobin, Hb E. At first sight, this is a straightforward missense mutation in which a GAG→AAG change at codon 26 of the first exon of the β-globin gene substitutes lysine for glutamic acid (Fig. 4.17). However, it also creates a cryptic donor splice site that competes with the normal donor splice site at the start of intron 1. Some 40% of splice events use the cryptic site, creating a truncated first exon and an out-of-frame junction with exon 2. There is no detectable β-globin product from this abnormally spliced mRNA and Hb E is thus synthesized at only 60% of its normal level.

The four classes of RNA splicing mutations – splice junction changes, consensus region changes, internal intron changes and the activation of cryptic sites – illustrate the complexities of the precise removal of introns. Amongst the β-thalassaemia syndromes they account for almost one-third of all mutations. Examples of similar mutations are beginning to emerge in other Mendelian disorders.

Normally spliced RNA from β gene

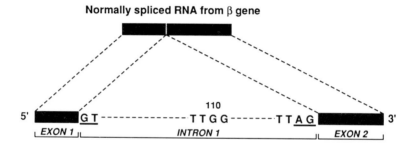

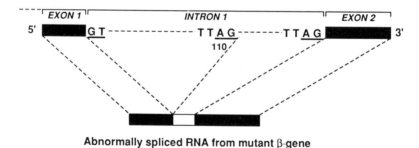

Abnormally spliced RNA from mutant β-gene

Fig. 4.16. Alternative splicing of the first intron of the β-globin gene. A G→A substitution at position 110 in intron 1 creates a new acceptor site that mimics the correct acceptor site. When the new acceptor is used in splicing, the resulting mature mRNA contains an additional 19 nucleotides of intron sequence (shown as the open box), and this causes a frameshift in exon 2. Only part of the β-globin gene is shown in this diagram.

Codon no.	24	25	26	27
Normal β-gene	GGT	GGT	GAG	GCC
Normal β-globin	gly	gly	glu	ala
β^E-Gene	GGT	GGT	<u>AAG</u>	GCC
β^E-Globin	gly	gly	lys	ala
β-Gene donor site (intron 1)		GTTGG		
Consensus donor site		GT $\overset{\text{A}}{\underset{\text{G}}{}}$ AG		

Fig. 4.17. Creation of a cryptic donor site by a point mutation in codon 26 of exon 1 of the β-globin gene. The GAG→AAG change in codon 26 substitutes lysine for glutamic acid in Hb E. It also creates a new donor site for splicing, GTAAG (underlined). Although the normal donor site in intron 1 of the β-globin gene is GTTGG, other favoured (or consensus) donor sites are GTAAG and GTGAG. Some 40% of splice events in the β^E-gene use the new donor site and thus part of exon 1 is removed. Furthermore, this abnormally spliced mRNA is out of frame in exon 2 and produces no detectable β-globin. The remaining 60% of splice events produce an RNA that differs from normal by a missense mutation in codon 26. This is the source of Hb E.

TRANSCRIPTIONAL MUTATIONS

It has been pointed out that blocks of DNA upstream from the 5′ end of the gene are involved in the regulation of transcription (see Fig. 3.6). Several point mutations have now been described in these promoter regions and confirm their importance in the control of the gene transcription. Amongst the various β-thalassaemic states there are now several involving point mutations in either the TATA box or the CACCC region further upstream. As expected, these reduce, but do not abolish, transcription, and the resulting phenotype is a β$^+$-thalassaemia.

MUTATIONS AND NORMAL VARIATION

The types of mutation discussed in the preceding section usually involve changes in the DNA encoding specific proteins and are therefore likely to have pathological consequences. However, as we have already seen, this is not inevitably the case. Synonymous mutations, particularly in the third base of a codon, may not alter the amino acid residue specified and will be genetically silent. Missense mutations that encode a different amino acid residue with properties similar to those of the replaced residue may have little effect on the functional properties of the resulting protein. Many genetic polymorphisms, discovered by analysis of protein differences between individuals, belong in this category. In the 1960s, Professor Harry Harris and his colleagues at the Galton Laboratory in London embarked on a systematic search for such protein polymorphisms, and concluded that in as many as one in three of the proteins they examined there was evidence for systematic normal variation in human populations.

The study of protein polymorphisms focuses on coding DNA, where mutations are subjected to the type of selection pressure that will rapidly eliminate disadvantageous genes. It is therefore perhaps unsurprising that, as techniques have evolved for studying non-coding DNA, the range of genetic variation in non-coding sequences has turned out to be very much greater. Two main types of sequence variation have emerged; point mutations and variable numbers of repeating units, and these are discussed below. How they are used in tracking genes is the subject of Chapter 5.

RESTRICTION FRAGMENT LENGTH POLYMORPHISMS

Restriction endonucleases have remarkable specificity and will not tolerate any changes in the sequence of bases representing the recognition site for cleavage. Point mutations can therefore abolish existing recognition sites, as well as create new ones. The consequence is the generation of a restriction fragment of altered length. In the example shown in Fig. 4.18, a restriction site present on chromosome A has been abolished by mutation on chromosome B. If DNA from an individual homozygous for chromosome A is digested with the restriction enzyme, Southern blotted and hybridized to an appropriate probe, the resulting fragments will be smaller (and therefore migrate further towards the anode) than the fragment seen in an individual homozygous for chromosome B. Heterozygotes will show all three fragments. If the recognition site variation is reasonably common amongst normal individuals it represents a polymorphism, and since it is recognized by the length of the fragments it is called a restriction fragment length polymorphism or RFLP.

Point mutations in DNA, particularly in non-coding regions, occur about once in every 100 to 150 bases in the genome, and one in six random base changes creates or destroys a restriction site. One may therefore expect to find an RFLP at least once in every kilobase-pair of DNA. The recognition sites of *Taq*I (TCGA) and *Msp*I (CCGG) show a higher degree of polymorphism than those of other restriction enzymes, probably because the dinucleotide CG is particularly prone to mutation. RFLPs are stably inherited as Mendelian codominants. Their main limitation is that only two alleles are possible, corresponding to the presence or absence of the restriction site. (It must be noted that the allele represented by chromosome A in Fig. 4.18 generates two fragments but is still a single allele.) Thus individuals in the population can be of only three genotypes, that is A/A, B/B or A/B, in this example.

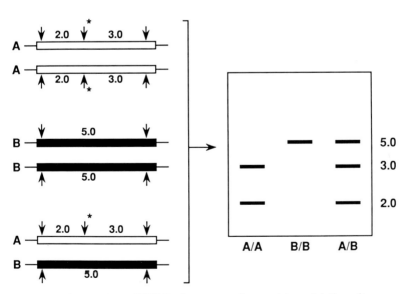

Fig. 4.18. Generation of RFLPs due to a polymorphic restriction site (arrows with asterisk) present on chromosomes A but not on chromosomes B. Southern blot patterns are shown on the right.

REPEATING UNIT POLYMORPHISMS

The relative limitation in informativeness of RFLPs is now being over-come by the discovery of a different type of sequence variation, in which blocks of DNA are repeated a variable number of times in different individuals. The first of these to be defined were short sequences of 9 to 70 bp, arranged head-to-tail in tandem array, and referred to as variable number of tandem repeats (VNTRs) or minisatellites. The number of repeats at a VNTR locus may vary, in different individuals, from a few copies to hundreds of copies, and such polymorphism can be detected by using a restriction enzyme that cuts outside the repeat region to give hybridizable fragments of different sizes (Fig. 4.19). In contrast to RFLPs, there are now large numbers of different genotypes, and a reasonable chance that two random individuals will be distinguishable. Although the basic repeat unit at each VNTR locus is different, several have an identical core sequence and it is thus possible to develop probes that recognize the repeat units at several VNTR loci simultaneously. This gives an enor-mous amount of inter-individual variability and is the basis of the technique of genetic fingerprinting (Fig. 4.20).

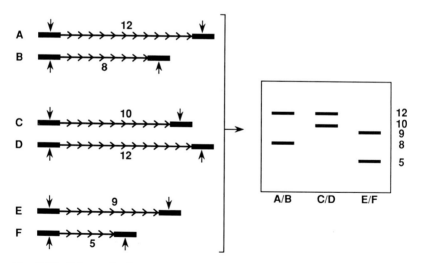

Fig. 4.19. Schematic illustration of VNTR polymorphism. The number of tandem repeat units is shown for a repeat-containing region of homologous pairs of chromosomes in three different individuals. Note that DNA from each individual should generate at most two bands on a Southern blot.

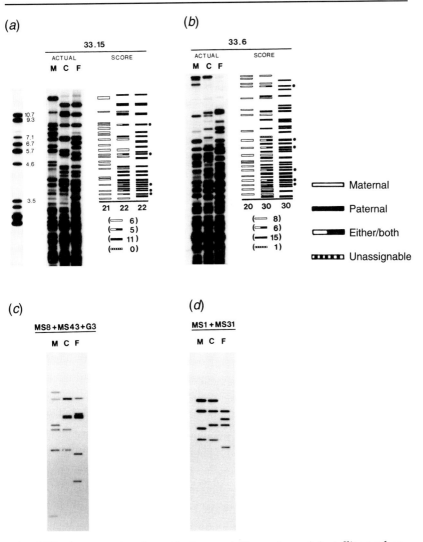

Fig. 4.20. An example of genetic fingerprinting using minisatellite probes that recognize VNTRs at several loci simultaneously. Each of the four blots shows band patterns in a mother (M), child (C) and putative father (F) with multi-locus probes (*a*) and (*b*) or combinations of single-locus probes (*c*) and (*d*). In (*a*) and (*b*) bands are scored as maternal, paternal, either/both or unassignable. The conclusion is that paternity has been established with the child having one new mutant band in (*b*). From Jeffreys *et al.* (1991). Copyright © by The American Society of Human Genetics. All rights reserved.

Another useful class of repeat unit polymorphism are the dinucleotide or CA repeats (also referred to as microsatellite or GT repeats). There may be as many as 50 000 blocks of CA repeats interspersed in the human genome, with a variable unit of 10 to 60 copies. Because the repeat unit is so small, this type of polymorphism is detected by PCR amplification of the block, and analysis on a polyacrylamide sequencing gel. Individuals that differ by a single CA dinucleotide can be detected quite easily (Fig 4.21).

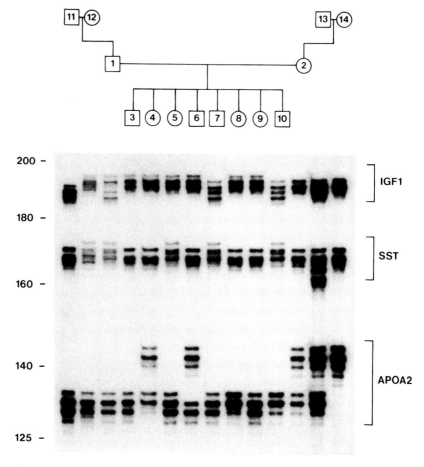

Fig. 4.21. An example of microsatellite typing of a large family at three separate loci (IGF1, SST, APOA2). Fragment sizes (bp) are marked at left. From Weber and May (1989). Copyright © by The American Society of Human Genetics. All rights reserved.

98

VNTR (minisatellite) and CA repeat (microsatellite) polymorphisms are currently the most widely used hypervariable systems for gene tracking (see Chapter 5). However, the human genome has other classes of repeat unit – such as alphoid repeats at chromosome centromeres and subtelomeric repeats at chromosome ends – that also play a part in genetic analysis. Furthermore, some repeats such as VNTRs also contain RFLPs within their tandem arrays and thus permit the description of quite staggering degrees of individual variability.

SUGGESTED READING

Antonarakis, S. E., Kazazian, H. H. and Orkin, S. H. (1985). DNA polymorphism and molecular pathology of the haemoglobin gene clusters. *Human Genetics* **69**: 1–14.

Antonarakis, S. E., Youssoufian, H. and Kazazian, H. H. (1987). Review: molecular genetics of haemophilia A in man. *Molecular and Biological Medicine* **4**: 81–94.

Brantly, M., Nukiwa, T. and Crystal, R. G. (1988). Molecular basis of alpha-1-antitrypsin deficiency. *American Journal of Medicine* **84**: 13–31.

Cooper, D. N. and Krawczak, M. (1991). Mechanisms of insertional mutagenesis in human genes causing genetic disease. *Human Genetics* **87**: 409–415.

Cooper, D. N. and Youssoufian, H. (1988). The CpG dinucleotide and human genetic disease. *Human Genetics* **78**: 151–155.

Darras, B. T. (1990). Molecular genetics of Duchenne and Becker muscular dystrophy. *Journal of Pediatrics* **117**: 1–15.

Hoffman, E. P. and Kunkel, L. M. (1989). Dystrophin abnormalities in Duchenne/Becker muscular dystrophy. *Neuron* **2**: 1019–1029.

Jeffreys, A. J., Neumann, R. and Wilson, V. (1990). Repeat unit sequence variation in mini-satellites: a novel source of DNA polymorphism for studying variation and mutation by single molecule analysis. *Cell* **60**: 473–485.

Jeffreys, A. J., Turner, M. and Debenham, P. (1991). The efficiency of multilocus DNA fingerprint probes for individualization and establishment of family relationships determined from extensive casework. *American Journal of Human Genetics* **48**: 824–840.

Jeffreys, A. J., Wilson, V. and Thein, S. L. (1985). Hypervariable "mini-satellite" regions in human DNA. *Nature (London)* **314**: 67–73.

Kazazian, H. H. (1990). The thalassaemia syndromes: molecular basis and prenatal diagnosis in 1990. *Seminars in Haematology* **27**: 209–228.

Kazazian, H. H. and Antonarakis, S. E. (1988). The varieties of mutation. In Childs, B., Holtzman, N. A., Kazazian, H. H. and Valle, D. L. (Editors), *Molecular Genetics in Medicine*. pp. 43–67, Elsevier, New York.

Kazazian, H. H. and Boehm, C. D. (1988). Molecular basis and prenatal diagnosis of β-thalassaemia. *Blood* **72**: 1107–1116.

Konecki, D. S. and Lichter-Konecki, U. (1991). The phenylketonuria locus: current knowledge about alleles and mutations of the phenylalanine hydroxylase gene in various populations. *Human Genetics* **87**: 377–388.

Piantanida, T. (1988). The molecular genetics of colour vision and colour blindness. *Trends in Genetics* **4**: 319–323.

Robertson, J., Ross, A. M. and Burgoyne, L. A. (Editors) (1990). *DNA in Forensic Science*. Ellis Horwood, New York.

Tsui, L.-C., Romeo, G., Greger, R. and Gorini, S. (Editors) (1991). *The Identification of the Cystic Fibrosis Gene*, Plenum Press, New York.

Tuddenham, E. G. D., Cooper, D. M., Gitschier, J., Higuchi, M., Hoyer, L. W., Yoshioka, A. (1991). Haemophilia A: database of nucleotide substitutions, deletions, insertions and rearrangements of the factor VIII gene. *Nucleic Acids Research* **19**: 4821–4833.

Weatherall, D. J. (1987). Molecular pathology of single gene disorders. *Journal of Clinical Pathology* **40**: 959–970.

Weber, J. L. and May, P. E. (1989). Abundant class of human DNA polymorphisms which can be typed using the polymerase chain reaction. *American Journal of Human Genetics* **44**: 388–396.

Zielenski, J. Markiewicz, D., Rininsland, F., Rommens, J. and Tsui, L.-C. (1991). A cluster of highly polymorphic dinucleotide repeats in intron 17B of the cystic fibrosis transmembrane conductance regulator gene. *American Journal of Human Genetics* **49**: 1256–1262.

5 GENE TRACKING

The preceding chapters, on the nature and extent of genetic diseases, on the range of technologies used in gene analysis, and on the mutational basis of normal and abnormal variation, provide a background for consideration of how this knowledge may be applied in the management of a range of genetic and partly genetic disorders. The term management is used deliberately. It is an unfortunate fact that genetic diseases cannot be cured, even though prospects of gene therapy offer some chance of this being a realizable goal in the not too distant future. Likewise, most genetic diseases cannot be even adequately treated, and in many of those that can (e.g. phenylketonuria, congenital hypothyroidism), therapeutic modes have developed in an ad hoc fashion largely independent of the exact molecular basis of the condition.

For these reasons, the major thrust of applied molecular genetics at present is in following mutant genes as they segregate in families and occasionally in whole populations. This endeavour has been termed gene tracking. Its main purpose is to give individuals and couples a better understanding of the chances of passing disease-causing genes to their offspring and to offer opportunities of avoiding this happening. Gene tracking is thus intimately connected with genetic counselling, and no applied molecular genetics laboratory can afford to operate in a scientific cocoon. Likewise no genetic counsellor can now afford to be ignorant of the ever widening scope, but still present limitations, of molecular genetic analysis.

As the following chapters show, molecular genetics has applications in a range of disorders not all of which show simple modes of transmission. However, its widest usefulness is where a mutant gene at a single genetic locus is entirely responsible for the pathology of a particular disorder. Tracking genes in Mendelian disorders is of immediate practical value in prenatal diagnosis, in presymptomatic diagnosis of late-onset, dominantly inherited conditions (such as Huntington's disease), and in carrier detection in both autosomal recessive and X-linked recessive diseases. It is also beginning to be used in confirming diagnoses in disorders in which clinical symptoms are ambiguous, and in establishing the prognosis in heterogeneous conditions associated with a wide range of possible severity.

PRINCIPLES OF DIRECT AND INDIRECT GENE TRACKING

Methods of gene tracking may be divided into two broad groups; the direct and the indirect (Table 5.1). Direct methods involve searching for specific mutant alleles at a particular genetic locus. Before this is possible, the normal gene will have had to be cloned and at least partly sequenced. Furthermore, it will be necessary to have quite extensive information on the exact nature of the mutant alleles comprising the disorder. Therefore any use of direct gene tracking must be preceded by an investigation of the range of mutational events that have been encountered (and continue to be discovered) in the disease in question. It is now apparent that virtually all Mendelian disorders are characterized by extensive heterogeneity. This means that although direct methods are often simple and quick they may be limited by the wide range of target mutant alleles that have to be covered in often separate analyses.

Indirect gene tracking is quite different in principle. It relies on genetic linkage, the tendency of segments of DNA that lie close together on a chromosome to stay together during meiosis, and thus to behave as a linked unit. Genetic linkage has been recognized and studied for many years. However, its power as an analytical tool has been revolutionized by recognition of the huge array of different types of DNA polymorphism in the human genome (Chapter 4). By now it is apparent that virtually all Mendelian disorders will be found to cosegregate with one or more DNA polymorphisms, even when the exact nature of the gene responsible for the disorder remains obscure. This aspect of gene tracking is discussed later. At this point it is worth pointing out that indirect gene tracking is used to follow genetic loci rather than genes themselves, and can thus be used not only to track unsolved Mendelian disorders but also solved Mendelian disorders where extensive genetic heterogeneity frustrates a direct approach.

DIRECT GENE TRACKING

In direct gene tracking, a search is made for the presence or absence of a specific mutant allele at a defined genetic locus. In principle, this is straightforward and results will be easy to understand and inter-

Table 5.1. *Direct and indirect gene tracking*

Method	Comments
Direct	Detection of presence or absence of a specific mutant allele at a genetic locus. Usually necessary to have information on DNA sequence differences between normal and mutant alleles
Indirect	Use of DNA polymorphisms to track mutant alleles segregating within a family. The same marker system will follow any mutant allele provided it is at the same genetic locus

pret. In practice, direct tracking is often complicated by the molecular heterogeneity of most Mendelian disorders, so that the demonstrated absence of one mutant allele may conceal the presence of a different mutant allele not detected by the analytical method used. Fortunately, for many of the important Mendelian disorders there are simplifying factors.

1 One particular defined mutation may predominate. In cystic fibrosis, the 3 bp deletion, ΔF_{508}, makes up some 50% to 80% of mutations and is obviously the first to be searched for. In α_1-antitrypsin deficiency, the Z and S mutant alleles are responsible for virtually all the pathology.
2 Some mutant alleles are found at high frequencies in particular ethnic groups. The point mutation at position 110 in intron one of the β-globin gene (see Fig. 4.16) accounts for some 80% of β-thalassaemic mutant alleles amongst Cypriots. Virtually all cases of Tay–Sachs disease in Ashkenazi Jews are caused by only two mutant alleles.
3 The genetic background of an individual may give a clue to the most probable mutant allele or alleles in a particular family. The background is defined by tightly linked DNA polymorphisms comprising the haplotype (see p. 129). For example, two of the most common mutant alleles responsible for phenylketonuria are usually found in association with specific haplotypes.
4 Methods have been developed, and continue to be developed, that allow for a simultaneous search for a

number of different mutant alleles. PCR technology, which amplifies a defined region of the gene, is an important part of this approach in that it provides an enriched source of DNA for further manipulations. Multiplex PCR, in which several segments of a gene are amplified simultaneously, further expands the possibilities of searching for several mutant alleles in one experiment.

MAJOR ALTERATIONS OF GENES

In major alterations, such as deletions, duplications and insertions, that affect genes, the size of the mutant allele is often changed in such a way that digested fragments will migrate on an agarose gel differently from digested fragments of the normal allele. Southern blotting of restriction enzyme digested DNA will detect the normal and mutant alleles at different positions on the resulting autoradiogram. In the extreme example of the type of complete gene deletion that characterizes the South-east Asian variety of α^0-thalassaemia, there will be no signal at all in the homozygous affected individual (see Fig. 3.15).

In a majority of disorders in which deletions are found, only part of the relevant gene is altered. This is illustrated by the Duchenne (DMD) and Becker (DMD) muscular dystrophies (see p. 79). Since the dystrophin gene is so large, it must be fractionated by appropriate restriction enzymes into units that are manageable on Southern blots, and then hybridized to a panel of genomic or cDNA probes representing the whole gene or the exon-containing sequences. For example, a HindIII digest of the dystrophin gene produces a set of some 65 genomic fragments, which can then be hybridized sequentially to nine cDNA probes covering all the exon-containing fragments. Although this is a tedious and time-consuming process, it does allow recognition of virtually all deletion mutations, which in turn represent 60% to 70% of DMD and BMD cases. A short-cut is to concentrate on cDNA probes that detect regions of the gene most prone to deletions (see p. 79). An example of this methodology is shown in Fig. 5.1.

POINT MUTATIONS

In more subtle gene alterations, such as point mutations and small deletions and insertions, hybridization of digested DNA to genomic or cDNA probes will not reveal any new band pattern on a Southern blot. Two general procedures are available for direct tracking of these mutations, each dependent on exact knowledge of the sequence change in the mutant allele. One of these techniques has already been described, namely the use of pairs of oligonucleotides as detecting reagents, one oligonucleotide being complementary to the normal sequence and the other to the mutant sequence. The short length of synthetic oligonucleotides gives them the specificity to recognize minor changes in genomic DNA sequences, in a way that is not possible with larger cDNA or genomic probes. An example of oligonucleotide probing for prenatal diagnosis of α_1-antitrypsin deficiency is shown in Fig. 5.2.

The other technique for direct detection of mutations employs the exquisite specificity of restriction enzyme digestion. Most restriction enzymes will not tolerate even a single base change in their recognition sequence and if a point mutation has altered this sequence they

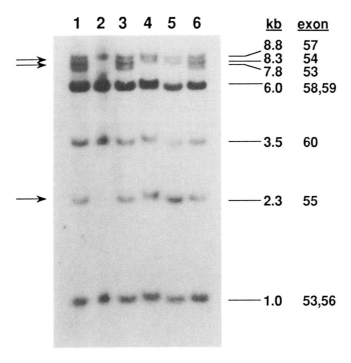

Fig. 5.1. Probing on a Southern blot for partial deletions in the dystrophin gene in BMD cases. Samples 1, 3 and 6 are normal male DNA. In samples 2, 4 and 5, part of exon 53 is deleted; in sample 2, exons 54 and 55 are also deleted. Courtesy of Dr Don Love.

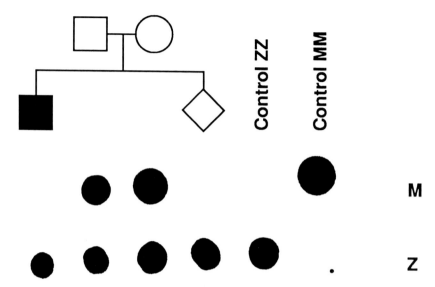

Fig. 5.2. Example of the use of oligonucleotide probing to carry out a prenatal diagnosis of α₁-antitrypsin deficiency. DNA from the four individuals in the pedigree and two controls is dotted onto a membrane and hybridized with M and Z oligonucleotide probes. DNAs in the index affected boy (filled square) and the at-risk fetus (diamond) hybridize to only the Z probe, indicating that both are homozygous for the mutant Z allele. In this and subsequent Figs, squares represent males, circles represent females and diamonds represent fetuses. Open symbols represent individuals of normal or unknown status, half-filled symbols represent heterozygotes and filled symbols represent affecteds. Courtesy of Dr I. McIntosh.

will no longer cleave the genomic DNA. Conversely, a point mutation may create a restriction enzyme site where before it did not exist. This point is illustrated nicely in the detection of three distinct mutations in exon 11 of the cystic fibrosis (CF) gene (Fig. 5.3). A sequence of 425 bp in this exon contains recognition sites for the enzymes DdeI (CTGAG) and HincII (GTCAAC). In the G1778→A mutation, known as S549N because serine (S) has been altered to asparagine (N), the DdeI site is abolished and DdeI will not cut this region. The digestion product is thus 425 bp in length rather than 174 bp+251 bp products generated from the normal gene. In both the C1789→T and G1784→A mutations the HincII site is abolished, and digestion of this region of exon 11 gives a single 425 bp product rather than 186 bp+239 bp products generated from the normal gene. However, in the G1784→A mutation a novel recognition site has been created for the enzyme MboI, and digestion leads to products of 182 bp+243 bp that are not produced by cleavage of the normal gene or of the two other mutations shown.

In both allele-specific oligonucleotide probing and also in differential restriction enzyme digestion, it is obviously necessary to know the exact sequence difference between normal and mutant alleles. Such information permits the design of PCR primers for selected amplification of the region being inspected. Therefore the types of analysis illustrated in Figs 5.2 and 5.3 are nearly always carried out on PCR-amplified genomic DNA. This increases the sensitivity and specificity of hybridization to oligonucleotides, and in the case of differential restriction enzyme digestion, removes the need for

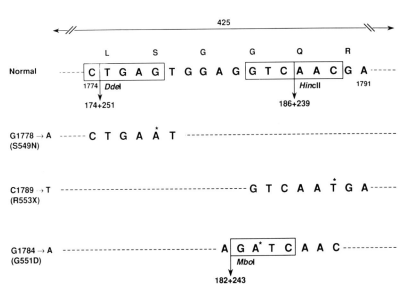

Fig. 5.3. Use of differential restriction enzyme digestion to detect mutations in exon 11 of the CF gene. The normal sequence contains recognition sites for DdeI and HincII (boxed sequences). In the S549N mutation, a G→A change abolishes the DdeI site and in R553X a C→T change abolishes the HincII site. In the G551D mutation, a G→A change also abolishes the HincII site, but simultaneously creates a new cleavage site for MboI. The mutated residues are marked with an asterisk.

hybridization completely. The amplified fragments can be visualized directly by ethidium-bromide staining of DNA resolved on gels.

SELECTIVE AMPLIFICATION

A method of gene analysis that is finding increasing favour in service laboratories because of its potential for automation is allele-specific amplification, better known by the more cumbersome title amplification refractory mutation system (ARMS). This is a PCR in which

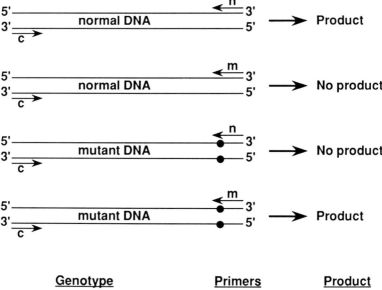

Genotype	Primers	Product
Homozygous or hemizygous normal	c + n c + m	yes no
Heterozygous	c + n c + m	yes yes
Homozygous or hemizygous mutant	c + n c + m	no yes

Fig. 5.4. Principle of the allele-specific amplification, or ARMS, technique. The common primer is marked by c, the normal primer by n and the mutant primer by m. Since it will not be known whether the target DNA is normal or mutant, two reactions are carried out, one having c and n primers and the other c and m primers.

two sets of primers are used, each set designed in such a way that it amplifies only either the normal or the mutant allele. Primers that mismatch with their target sequence by only a single nucleotide at their 3' ends will not amplify the DNA to which they anneal. It is obviously economical to have one primer common to both sets, and two unique primers known as the normal and the mutant primers (Fig. 5.4). Separate reactions are carried out and the amplification products inspected after gel electrophoresis and ethidium-bromide staining. In Fig. 5.5 the use of ARMS in detecting the ΔF_{508} cystic fibrosis mutation is shown, and compared to an alternative allele-specific hybridization procedure.

MULTIPLEXING

Multiplex DNA amplification or multiplexing is a procedure in which different DNA sequences are amplified by simultaneous PCRs. It is a powerful procedure for the initial examination of a case of DMD or BMD, since deletion-prone regions of the gene can be selected for amplification (Fig. 5.6). It is obviously important to ensure that each PCR generates a differently sized fragment, the presence or absence of which can then be visualized on an acrylamide gel. Multiplexing can also be conveniently coupled to the ARMS technique, which then permits simultaneous search for defined point mutations or small deletions. An example of the use of multiplex ARMS in detecting four of the more common mutations in the CF gene is shown in Fig. 5.7. In this case, each sample is examined in two duplex reactions, which permits better resolution of comparatively closely spaced bands.

EXAMINING mRNA

When genes are very large, even the most ambitious set of multiplex amplifications cannot cover the entire genomic sequence. In contrast, the mRNA transcripts of even giant genes are modestly sized (e.g. the DMD gene is 2500 kb and has an mRNA transcript of 14.7 kb), and thus more amenable to inspection for mutations affecting exons or splice site junctions. The difficulty is that abundant RNA is found only in tissues that express the disorder, and such tissues may not be accessible to the investigator.

It now seems probable that all tissues, whether formally defined as expressing or not expressing the gene product, have low levels of background mRNA for most, if not all, RNA species. This is referred to as illegitimate or ectopic transcription. It is not yet clear whether ectopically transcribed RNA is always correctly spliced and therefore identical with the RNA in an expressing tissue. None the less, it has

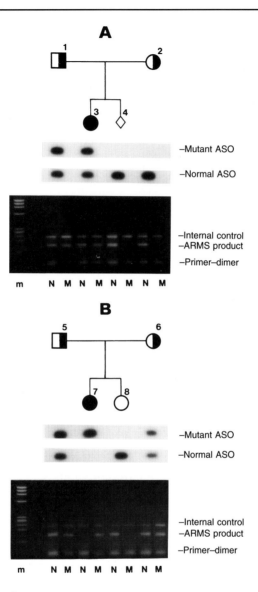

Fig. 5.5. Comparison of the ARMS technique and allele-specific
hybridization in detecting the ΔF_{508} mutation in CF. Immediately
below pedigree B is a series of dot blots hybridized to normal and
mutant allele-specific oligonucleotides (ASO). This shows the
affected child (7) to be homozygous for the mutant allele and the
normal child (8) to be homozygous for the normal allele. Both
parents are, as expected, heterozygotes. These results are

110

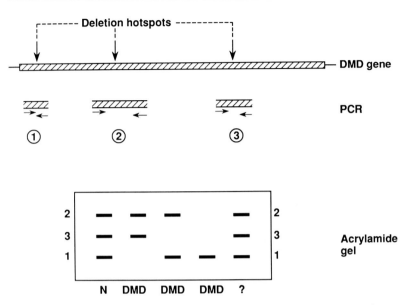

Fig. 5.6. Multiplex DNA amplification of regions of the DMD gene that are prone to deletions. Three (or more) different PCR reactions are carried out simultaneously, each designed to give a different-sized product. Absence of a PCR product on the resulting acrylamide gel indicates a deletion. However, a set of bands corresponding to the normal control (N) cannot be taken as evidence of normality, since this technique probes for deletions only in specific regions.

confirmed in the lower panel where the ARMS product from DNA of individual 7 is found only by using the mutant (M) primer and from DNA of individual 8 only by using the normal (N) primer. ARMS products are found with both N and M primers in the parents.

Pedigree A is more complicated. DNA from the affected child (3) reacts with both ASOs and gives ARMS products with both N and M primers. This means that she has inherited an unknown CF allele from her mother. However, since the fetus (4) has not inherited a ΔF_{508} allele from his/her father, he/she will not be affected with CF. See Fig. 5.2 for explanation of symbols. From Newton *et al.* (1990), with permission.

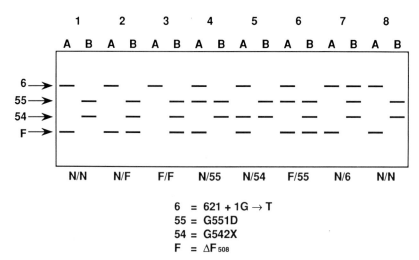

$6 = 621 + 1G \rightarrow T$
$55 = G551D$
$54 = G542X$
$F = \Delta F_{508}$

Fig. 5.7. Use of multiplex ARMS to detect four common CF mutations. Each sample is run in two reactions, A and B, and, in the absence of any mutation, the patterns shown in samples 1 and 8 are seen. The presence of G551D or G542X mutations is revealed by extra bands in reaction A, and the presence of ΔF_{508} or $621+1G\rightarrow T$ mutations by extra bands in reaction B. Note that in sample 3 the absence of a band in reaction A and an extra band in reaction B signals a homozygous ΔF_{508} mutation.

been possible to exploit ectopic transcription in characterizing several Mendelian disorders. The tiny amounts of specific mRNA from a non-expressing but accessible tissue such as lymphocytes are reverse transcribed into cDNA and thus examined by multiplex PCR (Fig. 5.8). This may well become the method of choice in searching for mutations in heterogeneous Mendelian disorders where the gene is large.

INDIRECT GENE TRACKING
Mendel's second law states that genes assort independently during meiosis, and that the behaviour of genes at one locus has no influence on the behaviour of genes at another locus. There is an important exception to this rule relating to genetic loci that are close together on the same chromosome. During the scrambling process in the first meiotic cycle, genes that are physically close together on a chromosome have a higher probability of staying together than do genes that

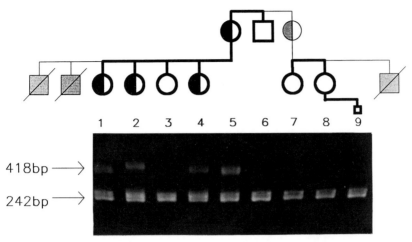

Fig. 5.8. PCR amplification of ectopic lymphocyte RNA to inspect for the presence of a DMD mutation in a family in which the disorder is segregating. Amplification of exon 17 is expected to yield a product of 242 bp. In the four females, 1, 2, 4 and 5, there is an additional band of 418 bp, showing that they are carriers of a tandem duplication known to be associated with a severe phenotype. The fetus 9 has not inherited this mutation. See Fig. 5.2 for explanation of symbols. Symbols that are scored through represent deceased individuals. From Roberts *et al.* (1990), with permission.

are far apart. This is illustrated in Fig. 5.9. Genes that tend to segregate together, rather than independently, during meiosis are said to be genetically linked (or more commonly, linked), and one set of such genes may be used to track another.

As so often happens in genetics, there are terminological traps in describing genetic linkage. In Fig. 5.9 it is the genetic loci that are linked rather than the genes themselves. However, most genetic loci are defined by the alternative genes, or alleles, found there and it is thus natural to use the term genetic linkage when the purist might demand the term locus linkage. In the sections that follow this convention will be followed. Occasionally, specific marker alleles are found that are linked to equally specific disease-causing alleles. This phenomenon is known variously as allele association, allele linkage or linkage disequilibrium, and is discussed on p. 127.

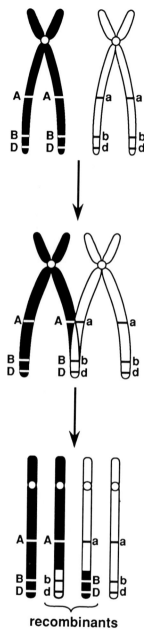

Fig. 5.9. Recombination (crossing-over) between homologous
chromosomes during meiosis. Three loci are shown, with alleles
A,a, B,b, D,d. This illustrates the principle that when loci are
physically well separated, alleles are more likely to recombine
than when loci are close together.

ESTABLISHMENT OF GENETIC LINKAGE

The establishment of linkage between two genetic loci in humans is a laborious and painstaking task involving a large number of observations on suitably structured families. It is essentially a statistical analysis of a set of reproductive events, in which the probability of alleles at one genetic locus cosegregating with alleles at another locus because the loci are close together on the same chromosome is compared to the probability that this has happened by chance. Usually one of the loci is chosen because it shows a suitable DNA polymorphism (the marker locus), while the other is a disease locus, which may or may not be occupied by a disease-causing allele (or alleles). The object of the analysis is to see whether or not the marker and disease loci are linked and, if they are, to get an estimate of the genetic distance between them. Obviously it is important to study families where there are a reasonable number of individuals affected with a particular disease.

In the two pedigrees shown in Fig. 5.10, the segregation of a dominantly inherited disorder, Huntington's disease (HD), is studied at the same time as the segregation of a DNA polymorphism that has four alleles, A, B, C and D. Inspection of family 1 shows that all the affected children and grandchildren of the proband I.1 have inherited allele A, while this allele is not found in the two unaffected children and the one unaffected grandchild. Much the same sequence of events is seen in family 2, but with one critical difference; the two affected individuals, II.4 and III.4 have inherited allele B from I.1. There are two possible explanations for these data. The marker locus and the HD locus may be close together on the same chromosome, so that allele A here cosegregates with the HD gene and only occasionally crosses-over or recombines as in II.4. Alternatively, the apparent cosegregation of marker locus and the HD locus is a coincidence.

In order to distinguish between coincidence and significance it is necessary to apply formal mathematics to linkage analysis. The probability of a set of observations representing true linkage is expressed as the logarithm (to base 10) of the odds, or lod score (Z). Lod scores must be calculated for a whole set of possible recombination fractions (θ), and represent the likelihood that two loci are linked at a given recombination fraction compared to the likelihood that they are not linked at all. Such calculations are complex and invariably involved computer programs such as MLINK or LIPED. A typical MLINK computer analysis of the pedigrees in Fig. 5.10 is shown in Table 5.2. In family 1, a maximum lod score of 2.12 is found at $\theta=0$, which is not

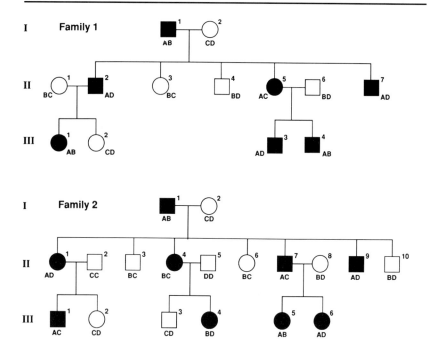

Fig. 5.10. Segregation of a dominantly inherited disorder, Huntington's disease, with a DNA polymorphism with four alleles, A, B, C and D. Filled symbols represent affected individuals; males are represented by squares, females by circles: In family 1, all affected individuals have inherited allele A from the grandfather, I.1. In family 2, two affected individuals (II.4, III.4) have inherited allele B from the grandfather, while other affected individuals have inherited allele A. There are two possible explanations for these findings: (a) the locus with the DNA polymorphism is linked to the Huntington's locus and II.4 is a recombinant and passes her recombinant chromosome to her daughter III.4; or (b) the apparent cosegregation is a coincidence. In Table 5.2, the probability that each of these explanations is correct is calculated.

surprising, since there are no recombinants in this family. In family 2, a maximum lod score is seen at $\theta=0.09$, which reflects the apparent recombinant chromosome in individual II.4, which is then transmitted without further recombination to III.4. Fortunately, given the comparatively small size of human families, lod scores for different sets of observations can be added together, so that the best analysis of this particular linkage is given by the column marked total. Here the maximum lod score is $Z=3.481$ at $\theta=0.05$.

116

Table 5.2. *Lod score analysis of segregation of HD and DNA markers in Fig. 5.10*

	Lod scores		
θ	Family 1	Family 2	Total
0	2.120	−3.918	−1.798
0.01	2.084	1.032	3.166
0.02	2.048	1.287	3.335
0.03	2.012	1.416	3.428
0.04	1.975	1.494	3.469
0.05	1.938	1.543	3.481
0.06	1.900	1.575	3.475
0.07	1.862	1.593	3.455
0.08	1.824	1.602	3.426
0.09	1.785	1.604	3.389
0.10	1.746	1.599	3.345
0.15	1.544	1.518	3.062
0.20	1.331	1.371	2.702
0.25	1.107	1.182	2.289

Positive lod scores are evidence of genetic linkage between loci, while negative lod scores indicate that linkage is less likely. Since lod scores are to base 10, a value of 3.0 represents a probability of 1000:1 that the observation did not occur by chance. Values of 3.0 or greater are conventionally taken as presumptive evidence of linkage, to be confirmed by further studies. The maximum lod score of 3.481 at $\theta=0.05$ from the data in Fig. 5.10 suggests a 3000:1 probability that the HD locus and the marker locus are close together on the same chromosome, but that recombination between the two might be expected in about 5% of meioses. The formal unit used to measure the recombination fraction is the centimorgan (cM), with 1 cM equal to 0.01, or 1% frequency of recombination.

Recombination fractions measure the genetic distance between loci and the probability of crossing-over during meiosis. There is a rough correlation between genetic distance and physical distance with 1 cM approximating 1000 kb or 1 megabase (Mb) of genomic DNA. There are many exceptions to this statement; male and female meioses often differ in the relationship between cM and Mb units, while at recombination hotspots 1 cM could represent considerably less than 1 Mb of

DNA. None the less, a 1% recombination rate or $1\,cM=1\,Mb$ of genomic DNA is a useful rule of thumb.

The example in Fig. 5.10 and Table 5.2 relates to the establishment of linkage between a dominantly inherited disease and a marker locus displaying multiple alleles. Similar calculations, though with slightly different assumptions, may be made for recessively inherited diseases and for marker loci with fewer, or more, alleles. Although the primary objective of such studies is usually to find a linkage, the exclusion of linkage indicated by a lod score of -2.0 or lower is also valuable. If the marker locus has a known chromosomal localization, then the disease locus can be excluded from that region of the chromosome. In this way an exclusion map of the human genome can be progressively built up, thus narrowing the remaining areas worth searching.

As the approximate chromosomal localizations of most DNA markers are either known or can be established rapidly by in situ hybridization, a positive linkage to a disease locus will usually place the disease gene in a moderately narrow region of a particular chromosome. The next step is to examine the cosegregation of the disease gene and other marker loci from the same region. Such multi-locus linkage analysis will eventually build up a genetic map of the region and, if suitable recombinants are found, establish the relation-ship of the marker loci to one another and to the disease locus. This is an essential stage in attempting to clone genes of unknown function by the procedure of reverse genetics. But it also serves the purposes of indirect gene tracking, particularly when marker loci are found that bracket the disease locus. A genetic map of the region surrounding the CF locus, built up by painstaking analysis of recombinants, is shown in Fig. 5.11. Note that there are sets of markers on both the centromeric and telomeric sides of the locus.

USE OF LINKED MARKERS IN INDIRECT GENE TRACKING

The data in Fig. 5.10 were used to show that there is a marker locus with four alleles that cosegregates with the HD locus. This locus, known as D4S10 and defined by a DNA probe G8, was used to localize the HD locus on the short arm of chromosome 4. A more detailed breakdown of part of the pedigree of family 1 is shown in Fig. 5.12, and indicates why allele A tended to track the HD gene. Because the two loci are close together, allele A and the HD gene operate as a tight unit during meiosis and are separated only

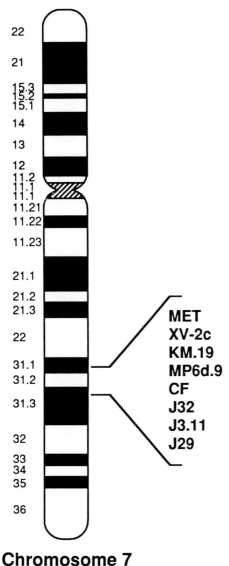

MET
XV-2c
KM.19
MP6d.9
CF
J32
J3.11
J29

Chromosome 7

Fig. 5.11. A genetic map of the region surrounding the CF locus, constructed by analysis of recombinant events, on a representation of the banding pattern of chromosome 7.

occasionally by recombination. They are said to be in linkage phase, or more simply, in phase.

An important point must be made about linkage phase. Although in both the families in Fig. 5.10, allele A was in phase with the HD gene, there is no prior expectation that the same situation would be encountered in any other family in which this gene is segregating. The marker allele could be A, B, C or D. Thus, in indirect gene tracking the first requirement is always to establish the phase relationship between allele and marker. The amount of information needed to do this depends on the mode of inheritance of the particular disorder and is best illustrated by specific examples.

In a dominantly inherited disorder it is normally necessary to study two affected individuals in the same family to be sure of the phase of the marker. This is illustrated in Fig. 5.13, using a simple RFLP with two alleles that are named by the fragment lengths determined from a Southern blot. The two affected individuals can be in different generations (Fig. 5.13a) or in the same generation (Fig. 5.13b). Sometimes one of the affected individuals is unavailable for typing, but the phase of the markers can still be inferred by difference (Fig. 5.13c). Note that this is the minimum information required, and a great deal more confidence that the phase assignment is correct is gained when there

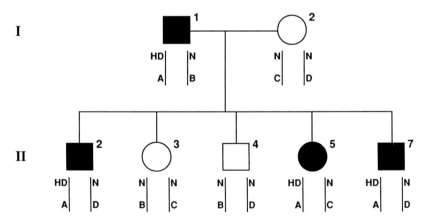

Fig. 5.12. A more detailed examination of part of the pedigree of family 1 shown in Figure 5.10. Allele A is on the same chromosome as the Huntington's disease (HD) gene, and the two loci are sufficiently close to remain linked in the majority of meioses. See Fig. 5.2 for a description of symbols.

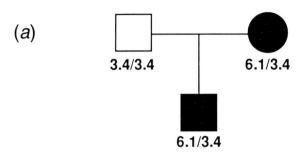

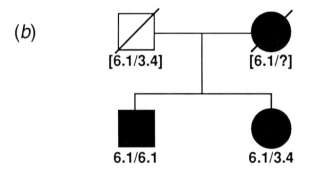

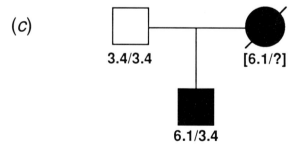

Fig. 5.13. Establishment of linkage phase for a dominantly inherited disorder and a tightly linked RFLP expressed as two alleles of sizes 6.1 and 3.4 kb. In each of the three pedigrees, the disease gene is on the same chromosome as the 6.1 kb allele. Inferred genotypes are shown in square brackets. Note that this is the minimum information needed to establish linkage phase. See Fig. 5.2 for a description of symbols.

are other affected (and unaffected) individuals in the same family
who are available for typing.

In an autosomal recessive disorder, phase is usually established
from a single affected individual and the two unaffected parents.
Each parent contributes a chromosome carrying the disease allele and
thus it is essential to be able to distinguish the parental chromosomes
(Fig. 5.14a). Sometimes this is not possible. In Fig. 5.14b, the affected
child has inherited a 2.1 kb fragment from one parent and a 1.4 kb
fragment from the other, but it is not clear which fragment has come
from whom. Thus, if a prenatal diagnosis were required in the family
in Fig. 5.14b, a 2.1/1.4 genotype in the fetus would indicate either a
homozygous affected or a homozygous normal. A 2.1/2.1 or a 1.4/1.4

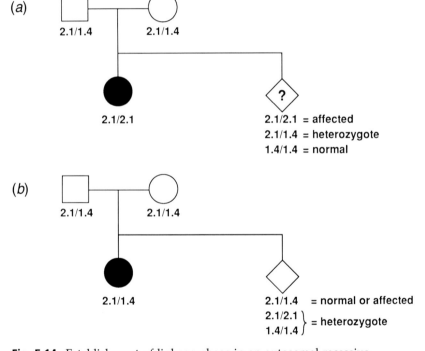

Fig. 5.14. Establishment of linkage phase in an autosomal recessive
disorder. The two-allele RFLP is expressed as fragment sizes of 2.1
and 1.4 kb. (a) This is a fully informative pedigree and the
genotype of the fetus can be deduced with certainty from the
band patterns. (b) A half-informative pedigree; the band pattern
2.1/1.4, which occurs on average in half of the fetuses, is
ambiguous. See Fig. 5.2 for a description of symbols.

genotype would signal a heterozygous, and therefore unaffected, fetus. This family situation is called half informative, because in only half of the cases is a definitive diagnosis possible.

Linkage analysis of X-linked recessives may be complicated by new mutations and by germinal mosaicism seen in these disorders. In the absence of such complications, disease-causing alleles can be tracked in a manner similar to that used for autosomal recessives. The difference is that males have a single X chromosome and this is inherited from their mother. The pedigree in Fig. 5.15 shows that it is possible to carry out prenatal diagnosis in an X-linked recessive using data from a single affected individual. Note that the band pattern on a Southern blot can also distinguish male and female fetuses, but only by different intensities in the 5.8 kb band.

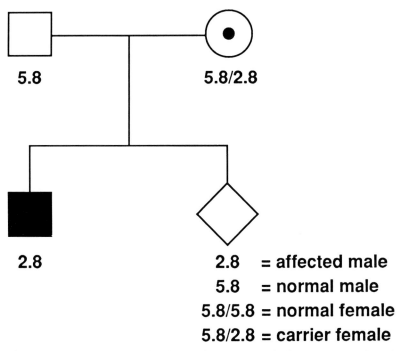

5.8   **5.8/2.8**

2.8

2.8   = affected male
5.8   = normal male
5.8/5.8 = normal female
5.8/2.8 = carrier female

Fig. 5.15. Establishment of linkage phase in an X-linked recessive disorder. Provided that the affected male child does not represent a new mutation, the fetal genotypes may be deduced from the band patterns of the linked RFLP. ⊙ represents a carrier female. See Fig. 5.2 for an explanation of other symbols.

INFORMATIVENESS OF DNA POLYMORPHISMS

In the examples given in Fig. 5.13 to 5.15, illustrative markers were chosen so as to be informative. In each case, key individuals were heterozygous for the DNA polymorphism so that the chromosome carrying the disease allele could be distinguished from the normal chromosome. The chances of this happening in practice depend on the nature of the polymorphism – whether it has two alleles or multiple alleles – and on the frequency of the alleles. For an RFLP with two alleles, the chance of any individual being heterozygous is derived from the Hardy–Weinberg equilibrium (see p. 11), and is $2pq$, where p and q are the respective frequencies of the two alleles. Maximum degree of heterozygosity occurs when $p=q=0.5$, but is still only 0.5, or 50%. Multiple alleles with evenly divided frequencies increase the chance of heterozygosity and a polymorphism with five alleles each at a frequency of 0.2 would give a degree of heterozygosity of 0.8 or 80%.

Degree of heterozygosity does not give a particularly good estimate of the likelihood of a marker being informative in a family situation, although it is a useful start. It is also confounded when particular marker alleles are associated with particular disease alleles (see Linkage disequilibrium, below). It is now becoming practice to use a different indicator of informativeness, the polymorphism information content (PIC). This is a mathematical formula showing the probability of identifying in any given offspring the parental chromosome contribution. For a two-allele system with frequencies of p and q, the PIC value is $1-(p^2+q^2)-(2p^2q^2)$; for a three-allele system with frequencies p, q and r it is $1-(p^2+q^2+r^2)-(2p^2q^2r^2)$, and so on. Thus if $p=q=0.5$, the PIC value is 0.375. Degree of heterozygosity overestimates the usefulness of markers for simple systems, but in multi-allelic polymorphisms, PIC values and heterozygosity tend to converge.

It will be obvious from the preceding remarks that finding suitable markers to track disease genes in a family at risk is not always easy. It is essentially an ad hoc process involving trial and error. Using markers with high PIC values to search for heterozygosity in key members of the family is a good starting point. Often the combined information from two different markers will solve a difficult problem. This is illustrated in Fig. 5.16, where each of the two markers is incompletely informative, but where use of both makes a prenatal diagnosis possible.

124

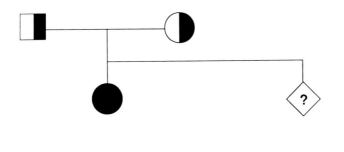

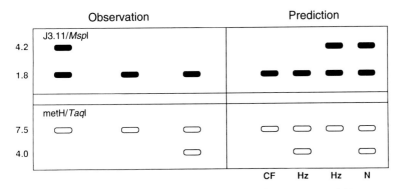

Fig. 5.16. The use of two different markers systems to gain full information on a family at risk of having a child with CF. In one system (J3.11/*Msp*I) the index affected child is identical with her mother, while in the other (metH/*Taq*I) she is identical with her father. By combining the two systems (which usually means running two separate Southern blots), a unique pattern is found for an affected child (CF), the two different types of heterozygote (Hz) and the unaffected homozygote (N). See Fig. 5.2 for an explanation of symbols.

ERRORS IN INDIRECT GENE TRACKING

The possibility of recombination between alleles at a marker locus and alleles at a disease locus places a limit on the accuracy of indirect gene tracking. If the recombination fraction is 0.05 (5% recombination rate) then the maximum accuracy of diagnosis is only 95%. In practice, the true accuracy may be substantially less than 95%, because in many families several meioses (each with a 5% chance of recombination) must be taken into account in constructing informative haplotypes. Calculations of error rates can become extremely complex, particularly when data on allele frequencies are included so they are usually carried out by computer programs such as MLINK.

A way of reducing the error rates associated with recombination is to use flanking markers, one or more polymorphic sites on either side of the disease locus. In this way it is possible to inspect directly for the possibility of recombination rather than using general odds on the possibility of such an event (Fig. 5.17). Only double recombinants

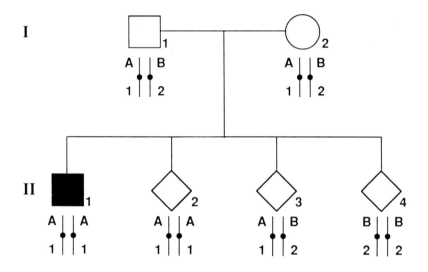

Probability of being affected (%)

	One marker only	Both markers
II.2	96.08	99.66
II.3	1.94	0.03
II.4	0.04	~0

Fig. 5.17. Example of error rates using linked markers to carry out a prenatal diagnosis of CF. In the hypothetical pedigree, two different RFLPs flank the CF locus (●), one system having alleles A and B and the other alleles 1 and 2. Each marker locus has a recombination rate with the CF locus of 1%. The probability of each fetus being affected is calculated for one marker system or for both marker systems. See Fig. 5.2 for an explanation of symbols.

could upset the diagnoses in such cases, and the odds on that happening are the product of the individual recombination rates, and therefore very low.

INTRAGENIC MARKERS

So far I have considered indirect gene tracking as a procedure in which alleles at a marker locus are used to gain information on alleles at a separate and distinct disease locus. However, there is no reason, in principle, why the marker and disease loci should not be the same. Most human genes are interrupted by intervening sequences of non-coding DNA and these regions are prone to mutation and the fixing of harmless DNA polymorphisms. Clearly, if such polymorphisms are used to track the coding part of the gene surrounding them, the chance of recombination (except for very large genes) is negligible.

Fig. 5.18 is an example of the use of an intragenic polymorphism to track the CF gene in a pregnancy at risk. PCR amplification of intron 17b reveals a highly polymorphic region of TA and CA repeats so that few unrelated individuals are identical. More than 25 different length variations have been detected in different individuals. In the example shown, the father and mother of the affected child have different band patterns, and thus it is possible to deduce the band associated with each CF chromosome. It must be noted that although a portion of the CF gene is being examined on the acrylamide gel, this is *not* an example of direct gene tracking, and information is always required from an index affected child. No data on the precise nature of the CF mutation is revealed.

The use of intragenic polymorphisms goes some way towards resolving the problems caused by errors resulting from recombination. It is also a valuable tool for dealing with disorders where molecular heterogeneity prevents direct analysis of the gene. However, as with all forms of indirect gene tracking, it is limited by the informativeness of the polymorphism used and by the need to test at least one index affected case to establish linkage phase.

LINKAGE DISEQUILIBRIUM

In the discussion of phase determination in tracking Huntington's disease, it was pointed out that there was no prior expectation of any particular allele at the D4S10 marker locus being on the same chromosome as the HD allele. This is not always the case for other markers and other diseases. If a disease-causing mutation has occurred comparatively recently, or if marker and disease loci are very close together, some marker alleles may be found to be associated preferen-

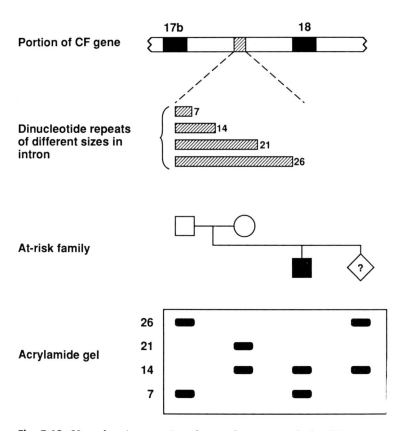

Fig. 5.18. Use of an intragenic polymorphism to track the CF gene in a family at risk. The intervening sequence between exons 17b and 18 contains a region of dinucleotide repeats that is so polymorphic that this repeat region varies in size between unrelated individuals. If this region is expanded by PCR and examined on an acrylamide gel, many different patterns will be seen in an outbred population, though no individual will show more than two bands. In the example shown, the CF gene is being tracked by this intragenic polymorphism, and the fetus at risk will be scored as a heterozygote. Note that although a part of the CF gene is being examined, this is still an example of indirect gene tracking, since the essential information is derived from the band pattern in an index affected child (filled box in pedigree).

tially with disease alleles. This is known as linkage disequilibrium or allele association and has some limited value in indirect gene tracking. Linkage disequilibrium is not restricted to combinations of marker and disease alleles and can occur at any set of closely linked loci.

It is important not to confuse linkage and linkage disequilibrium. If we return to Fig. 5.10, we note that in both families marker allele A was on the same chromosome as the HD gene (apart from the two recombinant exceptions in family 2). If we examined more HD families and continued to find marker A in phase with the HD gene this would be evidence for linkage disequilibrium. But this is not the case, and marker alleles B, C and D are found on chromosomes with the HD gene as often as they are found on normal chromosomes. Thus, although the D4S10 marker locus is genetically linked to the HD locus (linkage), there is no evidence for preferential association of alleles at these loci (linkage disequilibrium).

An example of linkage disequilibrium that has been of some value in genetic counselling has been described for CF. Two DNA probes, pXV-2c and pKM.19, define RFLPs at sites tightly linked to the CF locus. When DNA is digested with *Taq*I and probed with pXV-2c, polymorphic bands are seen at 2.1 kb and 1.4 kb. With *Pst*I and pKM.19 there are bands at 7.8 and 6.6 kb (Fig. 5.19). This allows for four possible allelic combinations or haplotypes on each chromosome 7, often referred to as A, B, C and D. In the absence of linkage disequilibrium, one would expect equal distributions of the four haplotypes on both normal chromosomes and on chromosomes carrying the mutant CF gene (conveniently referred to as CF chromosomes). Instead there is a preferential association of haplotype B with CF chromosomes (Table 5.3). This linkage disequilibrium is seen in all populations, although it is strongest in groups with a north European ancestry.

The linkage disequilibrium involving XV-2c and KM.19 has been used in genetic counselling to refine the risk of transmitting CF. It is of most value in advising couples where one partner is a known heterozygote and the other is of unknown status about their chance of conceiving an affected child. Without DNA typing of the unknown-status partner, a genetic counsellor would quote a risk of 1 in 100 ($\frac{1}{2} \times 1 \times \frac{1}{2} \times 1/25$), which is quite substantial because of the high heterozygote frequency (1 in 25) of CF in north European populations. If the unknown-status partner were typed for the ΔF_{508} deletion, and this found to be absent, the couple's risk would be reduced to about 1 in 400 (assuming ΔF_{508} accounts for three-quarters of CF

Table 5.3. *Haplotype distributions on CF and normal chromosomes in U.K. and U.S.A. populations*

Alleles (kb)		Haplotype	CF chromosomes (%)		Normal chromosomes (%)	
XV–2c	KM. 19		U.K.	U.S.A.	U.K.	U.S.A.
2.1	7.8	A	4	7	38	30
2.1	6.6	B	87	86	13	14
1.4	7.8	C	4	3	38	44
1.4	6.6	D	5	4	11	12

Note: Number of chromosomes scored: CF(U.K.) 884, CF(U.S.A.) 252, normal(U.K.) 874, normal(U.S.A.) 250.

mutations). Further refinement of risk can be achieved by examining the unknown-status partner's XV-2c and KM.19 band patterns. The carrier risks for individuals who lack the ΔF_{508} mutation are shown for the ten different XV-2c/KM.19 genotypes in Table 5.4. These risks may be applied to a variety of family situations. In the example

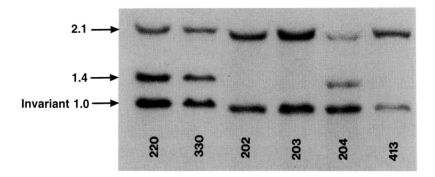

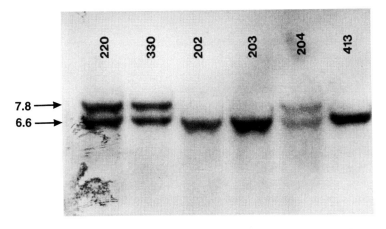

Fig. 5.19. An example of linkage disequilibrium with DNA markers at loci tightly linked to the CF locus. In the upper gel (XV-2c/*Pst*I system), the 2.1 kb allele is seen most often on chromosomes carrying the mutant CF gene. In the lower gel (KM.19/*Taq*I), the 6.6 kb allele is seen most often on chromosomes carrying the mutant CF gene. The haplotype 2.1/6.6, often referred to as the B haplotype, is found on about 85% of chromosomes carrying the mutant CF gene in the U.K. population (see Table 5.3). Samples 202, 203 and 413 are homozygous for this haplotype.

Table 5.4. *Odds that a random person of particular genotype and lacking* ΔF_{508} *is a CF heterozygote (U.K. data)*

Genotype	Probability	Odds
AA	0.00348	1 in 287
AB	0.02041	1 in 49
AC	0.00386	1 in 259
AD	0.00690	1 in 145
BB	0.03637	1 in 27.5
BC	0.02083	1 in 48
BD	0.02381	1 in 42
CC	0.00424	1 in 236
CD	0.00725	1 in 138
DD	0.01020	1 in 98

quoted above of a known carrier and an unknown-status partner who lacks ΔF_{508} but has an AA XV-2c/KM.19 genotype, the couple's risk would be about 1 in 900.

APPLICATION OF GENE TRACKING TO MORE COMMON MENDELIAN DISORDERS

In Chapter 2, Table 2.3 listed the more common Mendelian conditions found in the U.K. population. A reasonable test of the practical value of molecular genetics is to ask in how many of these conditions prenatal diagnosis and carrier detection can be based on either direct or indirect gene tracking. The answer is in a very high proportion; indeed there are only two exceptions in the list of 23. The current status of the major autosomal dominants, autosomal recessives and X-linked recessives is listed in Tables 5.5, 5.6 and 5.7. However, so rapid is the progress of molecular genetic technology that there is a reasonable prospect of further genes being cloned and additional linkages established by the time that this book is published.

Table 5.5. *Current status of major autosomal dominants*

Disorder	Chromosomal localization	Direct (D) and/or indirect (I) gene tracking
Familial combined hyperlipidaemia	11q23–q24	I
Familial hypercholesterolaemia	19p13.2–p13.1	Gene cloned (D + I)
Dominant otosclerosis	—	—
Adult polycystic kidney disease	16p13.3	I tracking (for major locus)
Multiple exostoses	—	—
Huntington's disease	4pter–p16.3	I
Neurofibromatosis type I	17q11.2	Gene cloned (D + I)
Myotonic dystrophy	19q13.2–q13.3	Gene cloned (D + I)
Congenital spherocytosis	8p21.1–p11.2	Gene cloned (D + I)
Polyposis coli	5q21–q22	Gene cloned (D + I)

Table 5.6. *Current status of major autosomal recessives*

Disorder	Chromosomal localization	Direct (D) and/or indirect (I) gene tracking
Cystic fibrosis	7q31–q32	Gene cloned (D + I)
α_1-Antitrypsin deficiency	14q32.1	Gene cloned (D + I)
Phenylketonuria	12q22–q24.2	Gene cloned (D + I)
Congenital adrenal hyperplasia	6p21.3	Gene cloned (D + I)
Spinal muscular atrophy	5q11.2–13.3	I
Sickle cell anaemia and β-thalassaemia	11p15.5	Gene cloned (D + I)

Table 5.7. *Current status of major X-linked recessives*

Disorder	Chromosomal localization	Direct (D) and/or indirect (I) gene tracking
Fragile X syndrome	Xq27.3	Gene cloned (D + I)
Duchenne and Becker muscular dystrophies	Xp21.3–p21.1	Gene cloned (D + I)
X-linked ichthyosis	Xp22.32	Gene cloned (D + I)
Haemophilia A	Xq28	Gene cloned (D + I)
Haemophilia B	Xq26.3–q27.1	Gene cloned (D + I)

SUGGESTED READING

Antonarakis, S. E. (1989). Diagnosis of genetic disorders at the DNA level. *New England Journal of Medicine* **320**: 153–163.

Berg, L. P., Wieland, K., Millar, D. S., Schlösser, M., Wagner, M., Kakkar, V. V., et al. (1990). Detection of a novel point mutation causing haemophilia A by PCR-direct sequencing of ectopically-transcribed factor VIII mRNA. *Human Genetics* **85**: 655–658.

Caskey, C. T. (1987). Disease diagnosis by recombinant DNA methods. *Science* **236**: 1223–1229.

Chalkley, G. and Harris, A. (1991). Lymphocyte mRNA as a resource of detection of mutations and polymorphisms in the CF gene. *Journal of Medical Genetics* **28**: 777–780.

Chamberlain, J. S., Gibbs, R. A., Ranier, J. E., Nguyen, P. N. and Caskey, C. T. (1988). Deletion screening of the Duchenne muscular dystrophy locus via multiplex DNA amplification. *Nucleic Acids Research* **16**: 11141–11155.

Chelly, J., Concordet, J.-P., Kaplan, J.-C. and Kahn, A. (1989). Illegitimate transcription: transcription of any gene in any cell type. *Proceedings of the National Academy of Sciences, U.S.A.* **86**: 2617–2621.

Chen, J., Penton, M. J., Morgan, G., Pearn, J. H. and Mackinlay, A. G. (1989). The use of field inversion gel electrophoresis for deletion detection in Duchenne muscular dystrophy. *American Journal of Human Genetics* **42**: 777–780.

Crystal, R. G. (1989). The alpha-1-antitrypsin gene and its deficiency states. *Trends in Genetics* **5**: 411–417.

Cutting, G. R., Kasch, L. M., Rosenstein, B. J., Zielinski, J., Tsui, L.-C., Antonarakis, S. E. and Kazazian, H. H. Jr. (1990). A cluster of cystic fibrosis mutations in the first nucleotide binding fold of the cystic fibrosis conductance regulator protein. *Nature (London)* **346**: 366–369.

Kerem, B. S., Zielinski, J., Markiewicz, D., Bozon, D., Gazit, E., Yahav, J., *et al.* (1990). Identification of mutations in regions corresponding to the two putative (ATP)-binding folds of the cystic fibrosis gene. *Proceedings of the National Academy Sciences, U.S.A.* **87**: 8447–8451.

Lalloz, M. R. A., McVey, J. H., Pattinson, J. K. and Tuddenham, E. G. D. (1991). Haemophilia A diagnosis by analysis of a hypervariable dinucleotide repeat within the factor VIII gene. *Lancet* **338**: 207–211.

Love, D. R., Flint, T. J., Marsden, R. F., Bloomfield, J. F., Daniels, R. J., Forrest, S. M., *et al.* (1990). Characterization of deletions in the dystrophin gene giving mild phenotypes. *American Journal of Medical Genetics* **37**: 136–142.

Malcolm S. (1990). Recent advances in the molecular analysis of inherited disease. *European Journal of Biochemistry* **194**: 317–321.

Newton, C. R., Graham, A., Heptinstall, L. E., Powell, S. J., Summers, C., Kalsheker, N., *et al.* (1989). Analysis of any point mutation in DNA: the amplification refractory mutation system (ARMS). *Nucleic Acids Research* **17**: 2503–2515.

Newton, C. R., Schwartz, M., Summers, C., Heptinstall, L. E., Graham, A., Smith, J. C., *et al.* (1990). Detection of ΔF_{508} deletion by amplification refractory mutation system. *Lancet* **335**: 1217–1219.

Ng, I. S. L., Pace, R., Richard, M. V., Kobayashi, K., Kerem, B., Tsui, L.-C. and Beaudet, A. L. (1991). Methods for analysis of multiple cystic fibrosis mutations. *Human Genetics* **87**: 613–617.

Ott, J. (1986). A short guide to linkage analysis. In Davies, K. E. (Editor) *Human Genetic Diseases: A Practical Approach*, pp. 19–32, IRL Press, Oxford.

Phillips, J. A. (1988). Clinical applications of gene mapping and diagnosis. In Childs, B., Holtsman, N. A., Kazazian, H. H. and Valle, D. L. (Editors), *Molecular Genetics in Medicine*, pp. 68–99, Elsevier, New York.

Roberts, R. G., Bently, D. R., Barby, T. F. M., Manners, E. and Bobrow, M. (1990). Direct diagnosis of carriers of Duchenne and Becker muscular dystrophy by amplification of lymphocyte RNA. *Lancet* **336**: 1523–1526.

Wright, A. F. (1986). DNA analysis in human disease. *Journal of Clinical Pathology* **39**: 1281–1295.

135

6 MOLECULAR GENETICS OF CANCER

Most cancers are not inherited, but occur as sporadic events in people who have little relevant family history. In the common human cancers the overall increased risk of malignancy in siblings of an affected individual is of the order of only two to three, a trivial factor and one of little use in genetic counselling. None the less, there are many reports in the literature of 'cancer families', where either several siblings have been affected or when an apparent autosomal dominant mode of inheritance can be inferred. Of course such familial aggregations could have a viral aetiology, or could simply be the result of chance, given that as many as 25% of Europeans and Americans can be expected to develop cancer during their lifetime. Alternatively, and as this chapter will attempt to show, 'genetic cancers' may provide a window to a better understanding of the origin of malignancy.

In recent years there has been a growing perception that most types of cancer involve changes in the genetic material at some stage of tumour formation. Two important pieces of evidence have been: (a) the observation that in many tumours there are cytogenetically visible abnormalities of chromosome structure and/or number; and (b) the discovery of cellular oncogenes and the mechanisms by which oncogene activation can contribute to carcinogenesis. These studies have been valuable in developing theories to explain tumour progression, but leave unanswered the question of whether the observed abnormalities represent primary or secondary mutational events. To address this issue, it is necessary to survey the inherited cancers, which, although encompassing probably fewer than 5% of all cases, are likely to provide important clues to the precipitating events. This concept is reinforced by the finding that for every inherited cancer there is a histologically indistinguishable counterpart that is non-hereditary.

136

INHERITED CANCERS

There are probably now well over 100 Mendelian conditions in which malignancy is a prominent (though not always inevitable) part of the phenotype. In comparison to the non-hereditary cancers, each of these conditions is individually rare. They may be divided into those with a dominant mode of inheritance and those that appear to be inherited as autosomal recessives.

DOMINANTLY INHERITED CANCERS

Examples of dominantly inherited cancers, several of which will be discussed later in the chapter, are listed in Table 6.1. For each of these there is a non-inherited or sporadic form that is currently clinically indistinguishable. However, the inherited syndromes often have an earlier age of onset and may be associated with multiple primary tumours. The principal tissues involved are listed, but in many of these cancer syndromes tumours may develop independently in other tissues, e.g. osteosarcomas in retinoblastoma, and small intestine, thyroid or liver carcinomas in familial adenomatous polyposis (FAP).

All these cancer syndromes are complicated by variable penetrance, expressivity and age of onset, which may make it difficult to distinguish between inherited and sporadic forms. In retinoblastoma and FAP, penetrance is high and tumour formation an almost inevitable consequence of inheritance of the predisposing gene. In contrast, although virtually all patients with NF-1 (Von Recklinghausen neurofibromatosis) have café-au-lait spots and neurofibromas, transition to full malignancy is very much less common. In multiple endocrine neoplasia type 2A, cancer develops in only 60% of the gene carriers by age 70. The Li–Fraumeni syndrome is characterized by such extraordinary tissue heterogeneity (see Table 6.5) that until recently there were doubts about whether it could truly be regarded as a syndrome. Thus the message of the dominantly inherited cancers is that, even though they may be expected to help in the search for predisposing mutant genes, these genes may be many in number and heterogeneous in function. This is reinforced by the different chromosomal locations of the cancer syndromes listed in Table 6.1.

RECESSIVELY INHERITED CANCER SYNDROMES

As long ago as 1874, Ferdinand von Hebra and Moritz Kaposi described a disorder in which affected patients developed skin tumours

137

Table 6.1. *Dominantly inherited cancer syndromes*

Syndrome	Principal tissue involved	Chromosomal localization
Von Hippel–Lindau	Kidney, haemangioblastoma of cerebellum	3p25
Familial adenomatous polyposis (FAP)	Colon	5q22
Multiple endocrine neoplasia, type 2A (MEN2A)	Thyroid C cells, adrenal medulla	10p11–q11
Wilms' tumour	Kidney	11p13–p15
Beckwith–Wiedemann	Kidney, adrenal cortex	11p15
Retinoblastoma	Retina	13q14.1
Li–Fraumeni	Multiple tissues	17p13.1
Neurofibromatosis type 1 (NF–1)	Skin	17q11.2

on sunlight-exposed parts of their bodies. This disorder, xeroderma pigmentosum (XP), was inherited as an autosomal recessive trait, characterized by extreme photosensitivity, a high incidence of cutaneous melanomas and frequent neurological abnormalities. Cultured skin fibroblasts from XP patients also have an increased level of chromosome aberrations when subjected to ultraviolet light or the action of chemical carcinogens.

The recessively inherited syndromes listed in Table 6.2 have three features in common: a predisposition to malignant disease, increased sensitivity to an environmental agent, and some form of spontaneous or induced chromosome abnormality. They are often referred to as chromosome-breakage disorders. In ataxia telangiectasia, Bloom syndrome, Fanconi anaemia and Nijmegen breakage syndrome, chromosome breaks are seen as spontaneous events in vivo. In contrast, there are no spontaneous chromosome abnormalities in XP.

The recessive nature of these syndromes suggested the likelihood of an abnormality in a specific enzymatic protein. It is now thought that most involve defects in cellular mechanisms for coping with environmentally induced DNA damage. DNA repair mechanisms are complex and may or may not involve prior excision of damaged

Table 6.2. *Recessively inherited cancer syndromes*

Disorder	Cancer risk	In vitro carcinogen – sensitivity
Ataxia telangiectasia	Leukaemia, lymphoma	Ionizing radiation
Bloom syndrome	Leukaemia, and other	Ultraviolet light
Fanconi anaemia	Leukaemia	Ionizing radiation
Nijmegen breakage syndrome	Lymphoma	Ionizing radiation, chemical
Xeroderma pigmentosum	Melanoma	Ultraviolet light, chemical

nucleotide bases. In XP there is evidence for an enzymatic defect in the DNA incision step that initiates the excision–repair pathway. However, complementation studies, in which cells from different XP patients were examined for their ability to correct one another's defects, suggest that there are at least seven separate groups, and force the conclusion that some seven different gene products are involved in this type of DNA repair. The genes responsible for the most common form of XP, XP group A, as well as that responsible for the rare XP group B, have recently been cloned. Different complementation groups have also been observed in cells from patients with ataxia telangiectasia. The rarity of the other syndromes in Table 6.2 has precluded complementation analysis, but there is clinical evidence that they may also be heterogeneous.

The study of Mendelian conditions commonly associated with cancer focuses attention on genes involved in rate-limiting steps in tumour initiation. It is clear that there are many different ways in which this can happen, and that both single genes (dominant inheritance) and pairs of homologous genes (recessive inheritance) can be involved. However, tumour initiation is only part of the complex pathway from normal to malignant cell. Even if the genetic alteration responsible for the initiating event has been identified, the susceptible cells must still progress through multiple steps (which may be reversible) to full malignancy. How this happens is still largely mysterious, but some important clues are beginning to emerge.

CANCER AS A CLONAL PHENOMENON

In theory, a tumour could arise either from an initial precipitating event in a single precursor cell or from a series of such events in a population of susceptible cells. The former would mean that tumours had a unicellular origin, usually referred to as monoclonal or just clonal. In the latter case, many cells would be responding simultaneously to the external precipitating event or events, and the

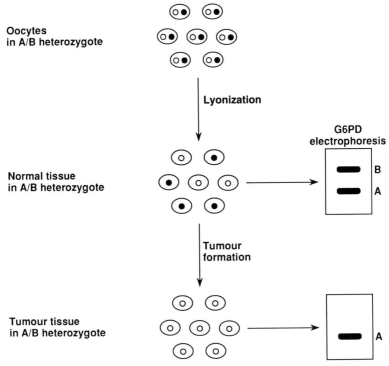

Fig. 6.1 Use of X-linked G6PD polymorphism to demonstrate clonality of a tumour. In oocytes, both X chromosomes are active in each cell (filled and open circles). After lyonization, normal tissue consists of a mosaic of cells, each cell having only one active X chromosome. Electrophoresis of the tissue shows both A and B isoenzymes of G6PD. If tumour tissue is available from a G6PD A/B heterozygote, it will show only one of the two isoenzymes (not necessarily A), since the tumour is derived from clonal growth of a single cell.

140

tumour would have a multicellular origin. This is referred to as polyclonal and pleoclonal. Following early work by D. Linder and S. Gartler in 1965 on uterine leiomyomas, it has now become clear that a very large majority of human cancers have a clonal origin.

Much of the best evidence for this conclusion comes from the analysis of polymorphisms coded for by genes on the X chromosome. As pointed out earlier (see p. 15), only one of the two X chromosomes in a female somatic cell is genetically active. X inactivation (lyonization) occurs at an early stage in embryonic life and is random, so that female tissues consist of a mosaic of cells, some expressing the paternally derived X chromosome and others expressing the maternally derived X chromosome. If normal tissue from a female who is heterozygous for an X-linked enzyme polymorphism such as glucose-6-phosphate dehydrogenase (G6PD) is examined, it will be found to display both alleles, since the tissue will be a mosaic of cells, some expressing the A allele and others the B allele. But if tumour tissue from the same individual is examined it nearly always displays a single allele, either A or B, but not both (Fig. 6.1). This leads to the conclusion that the initial precipitating event in tumour formation occurred in a single cell and was followed by clonal proliferation.

The G6PD A/B polymorphism has been used to examine the clonal origin of a number of different types of tumour. It is limited by the fact that the polymorphism is not found in all ethnic groups. It is also difficult always to be sure that a solid tumour does not contain non-tumour cells, and some early reports of pleoclonal tumour origins have had to be revised. It is now generally accepted that the only major exceptions to the unicellular, or clonal, origin of tumours are to be found in colon carcinoma, hereditary neurofibromatosis and hereditary trichoepitheliomas.

ONCOGENES

The clonal nature of most tumours suggests that mutation at a specific genetic locus might be an early event in the development of malignancy. The dominantly and recessively inherited cancer syndromes point to the involvement of many genes. However, inherited cancers are comparatively rare and may be misdirecting attention from alternative and more common mechanisms. The human genome is too large and complex for an undirected search for more prevalent cancer genes. Clues must therefore be sought in simpler systems. A major breakthrough was provided by analysis on an animal tumour virus, the Rous sarcoma virus, which as early as 1911 had been shown to induce cancer in chickens.

The Rous sarcoma virus belongs to a category of RNA viruses called retroviruses. On entering a host cell the retroviral RNA is copied into double-stranded DNA by a reverse transcriptase and then integrated into the host genome. Here it may lie quiescent, or be transcribed to produce multiple RNA copies of itself, or occasionally it may transform the host cell into a cancerous cell. An important clue to the generation of malignancy was the discovery of Rous sarcoma viral mutants that had lost their capacity for cellular transformation. Mutation had occurred in a viral gene named *src* which was thus implicated directly in tumour formation. However, the advent of molecular genetic technology established that *src* was not originally a viral gene, but rather had been picked up, or transduced, from host

RETROVIRUS

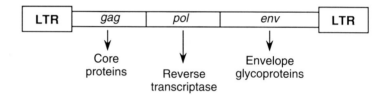

ONCOGENIC RETROVIRUS

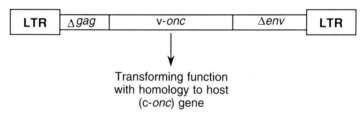

Fig. 6.2. Schematic representation of a retrovirus and an oncogenic retrovirus. The retrovirus contains genes responsible for production of core proteins, reverse transcriptase and envelope glycoproteins, as well as long terminal repeats (LTR), which assist integration and transcription. In many oncogenic retroviruses, genes responsible for viral replication have been partially deleted, but these viruses have picked up a gene (v-*onc*) from the host that, when expressed aberrantly by the retrovirus, causes transformation. The v-*onc* genes in the oncogenic virus are homologous to cellular oncogenes (c-*onc*) or proto-oncogenes.

cells in an earlier round of infection. This lead to a dramatic change in thinking and to the important concept that each viral oncogene (v-*onc*) has a normal cellular counterpart, the cellular oncogene (c-*onc*) or proto-oncogene (Fig. 6.2).

However, no tumour in humans has been shown to be caused by a retrovirus and thus the significance of proto-oncogenes in the development of malignancy remained in doubt. In the early 1980s, a number of investigators succeeded in developing transfection assays, in which fragmented DNA from human tumours was introduced into susceptible mouse cells in culture, and under appropriate conditions transformed the mouse cells into a malignant phenotype. Isolation of the transfected human DNA and establishment of the nucleotide sequence of the transforming gene showed it to be virtually identical with a particular retroviral oncogene, the v-H-*ras* gene from the rat sarcoma retrovirus (Fig. 6.3). This established that human proto-oncogenes were homologous to viral oncogenes and could be involved in the induction of cancer.

During the last few years many more proto-oncogenes have been identified, mainly from their presence in transforming retroviruses in animals. They have been highly conserved during evolution and are distributed ubiquitously in the animal kingdom. Clearly, proto-oncogenes are part of the routine cellular machinery, and under normal circumstances do not cause cancer. Integration of a proto-oncogene into the genome of a retrovirus is one mechanism of activation, but is probably of little significance in the induction of human cancers. The real importance of viral oncogenes is that they have provided an efficient mechanism for focusing on human proto-oncogenes that, through other mechanisms, are of major importance in the generation of tumours.

PROTO-ONCOGENE FUNCTION

That proto-oncogenes are found in normal cells and when disrupted can promote abnormal cell proliferation suggests a critical role for these genes in the control of cell growth and division. It now appears that the protein products of proto-oncogenes have key roles in the cellular signalling network and may be seen as relays in the biochemical circuitry that governs the behaviour of normal cells. Several classifications of proto-oncogene function have been made; that in Table 6.3 is not exhaustive, but highlights the major biochemical mechanisms by which these genes can act.

Several proto-oncogenes, such as *sis* and *int*-2, encode secreted growth factor proteins, which probably operate via autocrine loops to

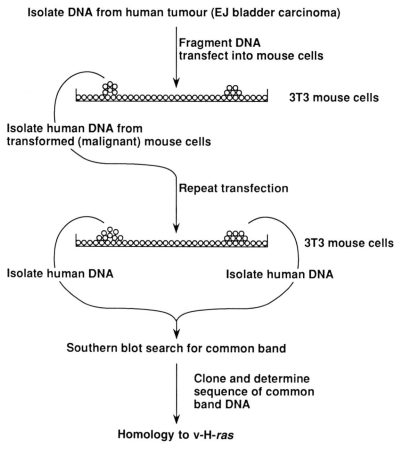

Isolate DNA from human tumour (EJ bladder carcinoma)

Fragment DNA
transfect into mouse cells

3T3 mouse cells

**Isolate human DNA from
transformed (malignant) mouse cells**

Repeat transfection

3T3 mouse cells

Isolate human DNA   **Isolate human DNA**

Southern blot search for common band

Clone and determine
sequence of common
band DNA

Homology to v-H-*ras*

Fig. 6.3. Transfection assay demonstrating that an oncogene in a human cancer has homology to a viral oncogene. The assay depends on transformation by human tumour DNA of susceptible mouse 3T3 cells, which then lose contact inhibition and pile up in visible foci. DNA is isolated from cells in the foci and used in the second or further rounds of transfection. DNA is then isolated from secondary foci and a human-specific probe is used to probe Southern blots for bands that are common to DNAs from the different foci. Cloning of DNA from a common band followed by sequencing showed homology of the human oncogene to a viral oncogene.

Table 6.3. *Function of some proto-oncogenes*

Proto-oncogene	Chromosomal localization	Protein product
Growth factor		
sis	22q13.1	Platelet-derived growth factor B
int2	11q13	Fibroblast growth factor
Growth factor receptor		
fms	5q34	Colony-stimulating factor receptor
erbB	7p11–p13	Epidermal growth factor receptor
Signal transduction		
src	20q12–q13	Tyrosine kinase activity
abl	9q34.1	Tyrosine kinase activity
H-*ras*	11p14.1	GTPase activity
K-*ras*	12p12.1	GTPase activity
Nuclear localization		
N-*myc*	2p23–p24	DNA-binding activity
fos	14q21–q31	DNA-binding activity

stimulate the growth of particular types of cell. Others, such as *fms* and *erb*B, encode growth factor receptors themselves, usually with intrinsic tyrosine kinase activity. A third large class of proto-onco-genes specify proteins that are involved in the delivery of signals from the surface of the cell to the cytoplasm. Within this class are genes that encode non-receptor tyrosine kinases (*src, abl*) and a family of membrane-associated G proteins, the GTP-binding GTPases, that couple growth factor and receptor interactions to second messengers in the cell (the *ras* group). The fourth class encode proteins found in the nucleus that have DNA-binding properties and are thought to mediate DNA transcription (N-*myc, fos*). This last group appear to act in cooperation with other classes of proto-oncogene product. Over 60 different proto-oncogenes are now known, and the list of functions in Table 6.3 is unlikely to be complete.

ACTIVATION OF PROTO-ONCOGENES
Since proto-oncogenes are normal cellular genes encoding proteins that are essential in cell growth and division, their participation in

oncogenesis is likely to follow some mutational event. A number of different mechanisms have been described for oncogene mutation. These are all somatic changes, characteristic of the tumour itself and not found in normal tissues of the same individual. Whether the somatic mutation is primary to tumour formation or whether it is secondary to other changes in the DNA of the susceptible cell is not yet clear, and it is probable that oncogene activation is only a part of the complex series of changes that occur in a cancer cell.

Point mutations

Normal mammalian cells contain three closely related *ras* proto-oncogenes, H-*ras*, K-*ras* and N-*ras*. They encode highly homologous proteins of 188 or 189 amino acid residues, the p21^{ras} proteins found on the inner surface of the plasma membrane. The p21^{ras} proteins bind guanosine nucleotides and have the ability to hydrolyse GTP to GDP.

Activation of the *ras* proto-oncogenes occurs by point mutation, predominantly, though not exclusively, at codons 12, 13 and 61. Substitution of amino acid residues in the p21 proteins reduces the capacity of the protein to hydrolyse GTP, and is thus thought to be responsible for unregulated cell proliferation. Individual *ras* proto-oncogene activation is dependent on tissue type; K-*ras* activation is found predominantly in colon, lung and pancreatic cancers, H-*ras* activation in bladder and urinary cancers, and N-*ras* activation in melanomas and haematopoietic malignancies.

Several techniques are available for rapid screening of tumour tissue for the presence of activated *ras* oncogenes. The most convenient is PCR amplification of the relevant exons in tumour DNA followed by probing with pairs of labelled oligonucleotides for the presence or absence of the appropriate nucleotide change (Fig. 6.4). In this way it could be demonstrated that about one-third of the samples of leukocyte DNA from patients with acute myeloid leukaemia contained point mutations in N-*ras*, predominantly a G→A transition in codon 12 of the gene. Specific codon 12 mutations of K-*ras* have been found in up to 95% of exocrine pancreatic carcinomas, and point mutations of H-*ras* in a variety of other tumour types.

Chromosomal translocations

One of the earliest examples of a consistent chromosomal abnormality in a tumour tissue was the Philadelphia (Ph) chromosome, found in about 95% of white cells in patients with chronic myeloid leukaemia. Although at first thought to be a deletion, it is now known that the Ph chromosome is a reciprocal translocation between the long arms of chromosomes 9 and 22, formally specified as t(9;22)(q34;q11). Molecular genetic analysis has revealed that the breakpoint at 9q34 not only disrupts the *abl* proto-oncogene (which has tyrosine kinase activity), but translocates it to the long arm of chromosome 22, where it comes under the control of a promoter region derived from 22q11, known as the breakpoint cluster region (*bcr*) (Fig. 6.5). The consequence of the translocation is the formation of a fusion gene, *bcr–abl*, that generates a new fusion RNA and

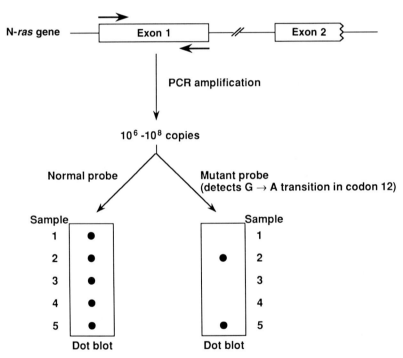

Fig. 6.4. Use of PCR amplification of exon 1 of the N–*ras* gene followed by oligonucleotide probing of dot blots to detect a point mutation in tumour tissue. The use of a pair of oligonucleotide probes will detect a specific nucleotide change. In this example, all five samples display the normal proto-oncogene sequence, while samples 2 and 5 show, in addition, the presence of a G→A transition in codon 12. To scan samples for the presence of other mutations in exon 1, further pairs of detecting oligonucleotides are necessary.

147

protein. The new fusion protein is larger than the normal product encoded by the *abl* proto-oncogene, and exhibits unregulated tyrosine kinase activity (also seen in the v-*abl* gene product). A similar translocation, also involving *abl* and *bcr*, is found in about 25% of cases of adult acute lymphocytic leukaemia, although the resulting fusion protein is somewhat smaller than that seen in chronic myeloid leukaemia.

The other major group of tumours in which chromosomal translocations have activated a proto-oncogene are the Burkitt lymphomas. The *myc* proto-oncogene is localized at 8q34 and encodes a product with DNA-binding properties. In the majority of Burkitt lymphomas there is a translocation between chromosomes 8 and 14, so that *myc* is moved to a point distal to the immunoglobulin heavy-chain locus at 14q32. In others *myc* is translocated to sites in either the kappa light-chain immunoglobulin gene at 2p11 or the lambda light-chain gene at 22q11. In these tumours the activated *myc* oncogene is expressed constitutively, perhaps because of structural changes in the normal negative regulatory elements in the first exon of the gene, or because of the presence of strong promoters or enhancers in the now adjacent immunoglobulin gene.

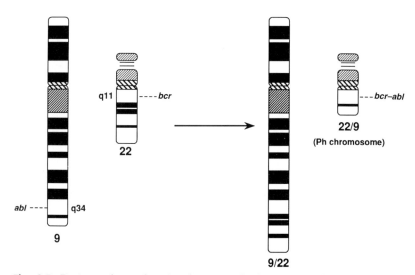

Fig. 6.5. Reciprocal translocation between the long arms of chromosome 9 and 22 to generate the Philadelphia (Ph) chromosome. The *abl* proto-oncogene is translocated from 9q34 to the q11 region of chromosome 22, where a new fusion gene *bcr–abl* is formed. This leads to activation of *abl*.

Gene amplification

Both cytogenetic and molecular studies have shown that some proto-oncogenes occur in multiple copies of tumour tissue. The *myc* proto-oncogenes are amplified in breast cancer, small cell cancer of the lung and in neuroblastomas, *erb*B1 is amplified in glioblastomas and *erb*B2 in breast cancer. The presence of multiple copies of the proto-onco-gene in a tumour often correlates with poor prognosis. In general, and within the limitations of restriction enzyme mapping, the proto-oncogene does not appear to be rearranged. Exactly how ampli-fication has occurred remains unknown. Amplification is obviously a mechanism whereby the amount and activity of a proto-oncogene product can be greatly increased.

TUMOUR-SUPPRESSOR GENES

Tumours arise when there is an inappropriate increase in the number of cells in a tissue. This could arise through a failure of differentiation, and in many haematopoietic malignancies there is evidence for pro-liferation of immature cell types that are blocked from moving into more appropriate pathways. However, the largest group of cancers in humans are those involving epithelial cells, where the problem appears to be one of unrestrained growth of an already specialized cell type. The discovery of oncogenes, and the growing understand-ing of their functional role in the cell, has therefore tended to focus attention on what might be called positive mechanisms for accelerated cell growth. The different mechanisms for proto-onco-gene activation – point mutations, chromosomal translocations and gene amplification – are thought to lead to gain-of-function changes that enhance the positive signals for cell growth. Although this is a crude and oversimplified picture, it has the virtue of drawing atten-tion to an alternative mechanism, loss-of-function mutations in sup-pressor genes whose normal role is to restrict undue cell proliferation.

The idea of tumour-suppressor genes has its origin in cell fusion experiments. When cells with a malignant phenotype are fused to cells with a non-malignant phenotype, the resulting hybrid is usually non-malignant, but may acquire a malignant phenotype on propaga-tion in culture as specific chromosomes are lost. This observation suggested that some chromosomes carry tumour-suppressor genes, and that either chromosome loss or loss-of-function mutations might lead to the emergence of a malignant phenotype.

There is an obvious difficulty in characterizing these putative tumour-suppressor genes. Transfection experiments (Fig. 6.3) allow

DNA sequences that have obvious transforming potential to be identified. The opposite experiment, in which a sequence that suppresses transformation is identified, is more difficult to design. Much of the evidence for tumour-suppressor genes comes from the finding that specific chromosomal regions are often deleted from the genome in tumour tissue, leading to the assumption that tumour-suppressor genes must be localized in these deleted regions. However, a more precise understanding of the nature of tumour-suppressor genes has been gained by molecular genetic analysis of some of the dominantly inherited cancer syndromes listed in Table 6.1.

RETINOBLASTOMA

Retinoblastoma is the most common intraocular cancer in young children with an incidence of about 1 in 20 000. More than half of the cases are sporadic and usually affect only one eye, with the tumours arising from a single focus. The remaining cases are familial, either arising as new germ-line mutations or inherited from an affected parent as an autosomal dominant. Familial cases usually involve multifocal tumours in both eyes, and are associated with a high incidence of other malignancies, of which osteosarcomas are the most prevalent. Dominantly inherited retinoblastoma has a penetrance of 90%, and thus tumour formation may occasionally skip a generation.

In 1971, A Knudson proposed a simple genetic explanation to account for the two different types of retinoblastoma (reviewed by Knudson, 1986). He suggested that all tumour cells in both types carried two mutant retinoblastoma (RB) genes. In familial retinoblastoma the first mutation was either inherited or occurred in the germ line, and was therefore present in all the cells of the body. If a second somatic mutation occurred in susceptible retinoblasts, the result was the formation of a retinoblastoma; if it occurred at a later time in another tissue, a different malignancy might develop. In contrast, in the sporadic non-familial cases both mutations occurred somatically and locally within a single retinoblast, whose descendents then expanded to form the tumour (Fig. 6.6).

Knudson's ideas were based on detailed analysis of the age of diagnosis of familial and non-familial cases of retinoblastoma, and the counting of the number of tumours per eye in bilateral cases. The data were consistent with a two-event model, and Knudson's two-hit hypothesis for tumorigenesis has been an important conceptual advance in cancer theory. It suggests that in familial retinoblastoma it is the susceptibility to the tumour that is inherited as a dominant (one mutant gene), but that the actual mechanism of tumour formation involves a second mutant gene and has therefore recessive expression. Occasional non-penetrance in familial cases would occur if no second mutation were suffered by the susceptible retinoblast. In sporadic cases where two separate somatic mutations must occur in a single retinal cell, unifocal tumours are the likely result.

The Knudson hypothesis also leads indirectly to the idea of a tumour-suppressor gene. In some familial retinoblastoma pedigrees, actual tumour formation can skip a generation and reappear in the progeny of unaffected cases. The fortunate escapees may inherit a mutant gene from a parent and pass it to their children, but without themselves incurring the second somatic event. It follows that a sin-

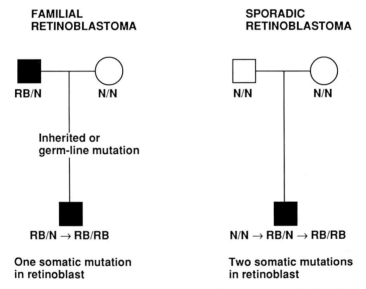

Fig. 6.6. Schematic representation of mutational events in familial and sporadic retinoblastoma. In familial cases, the mutant gene (RB) is inherited or created as a germ-line event and is present in single dose in all cells. A somatic mutation in retinal cells leads to retinoblastoma, whereas somatic mutations in other cells may lead to other malignancies. In sporadic cases, two somatic mutations must occur in the same retinal cell before retinoblastoma occurs. N represents the normal allele of the RB gene. In this and subsequent Figs, squares represent male individuals, circles represent females, filled symbols represent affected individuals, open symbols represent normal individuals (or unassigned individuals).

151

gle copy of a normal gene is sufficient to suppress tumour formation, and thus the normal retinoblastoma gene is the first of a growing list of tumour-suppressor genes.

Cytogenetic analysis of tumour tissue in sporadic cases of retinoblastoma revealed that in some cases there had been an interstitial deletion of part of the long arm of one of a pair of homologous chromosomes 13. The exact region deleted varied from one patient to another but usually involved band 13q14. This provided a localization for the RB gene and suggested that it could be inactivated both by deletions and by more subtle mutations. A genetic marker, the polymorphic enzyme esterase D, was also localized to 13q14 and could be used in linkage analysis to track the RB gene in familial cases. This analysis showed that the same gene was responsible for both sporadic and familial types of retinoblastoma.

Using molecular markers it has been possible to piece together the sequence of events that lead to tumour formation in a susceptible retinoblast. RFLPs that bracket the RB locus are available and these allow comparisons to be made between tumour and non-tumour tissue (Fig. 6.7). For purposes of illustration, it is assumed that a child has inherited one copy of a mutant gene (RB) from its parent and a normal gene (N) from its unaffected parent. It is further assumed that the chromosome carrying the RB gene carries a closely linked marker allele A and the chromosome carrying the normal gene carries allele B. All non-tumour tissue in the child would be heterozygous for A and B and would show a double band on a Southern blot. But if the normal chromosome had been lost in the tumour tissue, a single band, A, would be seen. The same would occur if there had been loss of the normal chromosome and reduplication of the RB chromosome, or if there had been mitotic crossing-over between normal and RB chromosomes, though in these cases band A would be more intense. Point mutation in the normal gene that generated an RB gene, or a small deletion involving the normal gene, would continue to show both bands in tumour tissue. All these events, and several others, have been observed in the pathology of retinoblastoma.

Using the existence of homozygous tumour deletions, the RB gene was cloned, identified and sequenced in 1987. It is a large gene, spanning some 200 kb of genomic DNA and producing an mRNA transcript of 4.7 kb. It encodes a phosphoprotein, with DNA-binding activity that is found in the cell nucleus. The gene appears to be expressed in virtually all tisues and mutant forms have been found in tumour tissue from malignancies other than retinoblastomas and osteosarcomas. There is now little doubt that removal of two copies of

152

the normal RB gene in retinal cells at an early development stage by one of the mechanisms illustrated in Fig. 6.7 is responsible for retinoblastoma. However, the involvement of the RB gene in other malignancies is probably more complex and is discussed below.

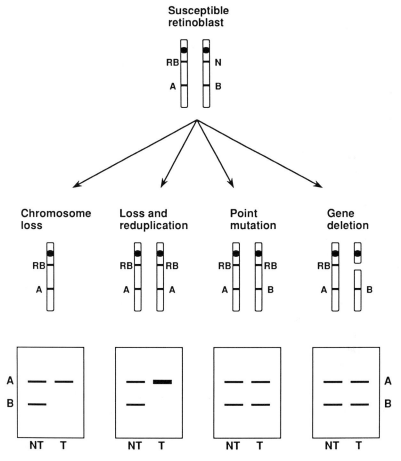

Fig. 6.7. Mechanisms by which a second hit on a susceptible retinoblast may result in retinoblastoma. The susceptible retinoblast may itself be the result of inheritance of a single RB gene, or may be derived from a first somatic mutation. The RB and normal (N) chromosomes are marked by alleles A and B, respectively. At the bottom of the diagram, schematic Southern blots of non-tumour (NT) and tumour (T) DNAs are compared.

WILMS' TUMOUR

Wilms' tumour, or nephroblastoma, is an embryonal malignancy of the kidney that affects about 1 in 10 000 infants and young children. Like retinoblastoma, it can occur in both sporadic and familial forms, although the latter are much less common than they are in retinoblastoma, leading Knudson to include it in elaborating his two-hit model of carcinogenesis. A subset of Wilms' tumour cases occurs in association with aniridia, genito-urinary abnormalities and mental retardation, known as the WAGR syndrome. Although familial cases of WAGR syndrome are rare, patients frequently have a cytogenetically detectable deletion in the short arm of chromosome 11 that has been mapped to 11p13. In sporadic cases of Wilms' tumour that are not associated with chromosome deletions, allele loss has also been observed on 11p. This observation suggested that loss or inactivation of a tumour-suppressor gene at 11p13 might be a primary event in the development of Wilms' tumour. By analogy with retinoblastoma, the first event in familial cases would be inherited and the second event a somatic mutation.

Molecular mapping experiments narrowed the location of the WAGR region to a specific interval in 11p13 bounded by the genes for erythrocyte catalase and the β-subunit of follicle-stimulating hormone. The map was refined by analyses of further constitutional deletions and by the discovery of the first tumour-specific homozygous deletion. Two independent groups, using different cloning technologies, separately isolated a candidate Wilms' tumour gene (WT1) in 1990. It encodes a 'zinc-finger' DNA-binding protein with an expected role in transcriptional regulation. In contrast to the retinoblastoma gene, the WT1 gene has a restricted pattern of expression, being found in mesenchymal buds, renal vesicle and glomerular epithelium of the embryonic kidney, fetal testis and ovary, and some haematopoietic cells. This may explain why mutation at the WT1 locus results in only one type of tumour.

It has become apparent, however, that the pathogenesis of Wilms' tumour is a great deal more complicated than that seen in retinoblastoma. In a majority of sporadic Wilms' tumour tissues examined, evidence for structurally or quantitatively abnormal RNA transcripts of the candidate WT1 gene is still lacking. There is, therefore, no compelling evidence that the loss of both copies of the tumour-suppressor gene at the candidate WT1 locus is in any way a complete explanation for tumour formation. Furthermore, study of the loss of heterozygosity (see below) of DNA markers at polymorphic loci on chromosome 11p in Wilms' tumours has shown that the most consistent losses occur in band 11p15, some 10 Mb distal to the region deleted in WAGR.

The possible involvement of a gene at 11p15 in Wilms' tumour is supported by finding in the Beckwith–Wiedemann syndrome (BWS). The clinical features are macroglossia, anterior wall defects, high birth weight, ear lobe grooves and hemihypertrophy, and predisposition to embryonal tumours such as Wilms' and adrenocortical carcinoma. A paternally derived small duplication of 11p15 has been found in several patients and BWS shows autosomal dominant inheritance with incomplete penetrance.

The complexities of Wilms' tumour do not necessarily invalidate the Knudson two-hit model of tumorigenesis. Probably only in retinoblastoma can it be seen in its simple form – the loss or inactivation of two copies of the same tumour-suppressor gene. In other cancers, including those with a clear familial aetiology, more than one suppressor gene is likely to be involved. It is tempting to conclude that, in at least some cases of Wilms' tumour, one of these may be the candidate Wilms' tumour gene at 11p13 and the other a gene at 11p15. However, there are families in which Wilms' tumour does not segregate with markers at either 11p13 or 11p15. Thus it is not yet possible to say how many genes are involved in Wilms' tumour nor can anything be said yet about the stepwise passage to a malignant cell.

SEARCHING FOR OTHER TUMOUR-SUPPRESSOR GENES

Studies on retinoblastoma and the WAGR syndrome, together with the cloning of the RB gene and a putative Wilms' tumour gene, suggest that clearly inherited cancer syndromes are a group of disorders worth analysing in the search for possible tumour-suppressor genes. If the disorder segregates as an autosomal dominant (even with reduced penetrance), batteries of polymorphic DNA markers can be used to track the susceptibility gene and to assign it to a chromosomal region. This approach has been used with success in mapping and cloning genes for several syndromes listed in Table 6.1 (e.g. FAP, NF-1).

However, most common cancers, even when showing familial aggregations, are not inherited in Mendelian fashion and are thus not susceptible to linkage analysis. An alternative approach is to search tumour tissue for the loss of specific chromosomal regions that, by analogy with deletions in retinoblastoma and Wilms' tumour, might harbour tumour-suppressor genes. The distributions of alleles at polymorphic DNA loci are compared in normal and tumour tissue from an affected individual. Since Southern blots do not lend themselves readily to quantitative analyses, a search is usually made for allele loss in the tumour of an individual whose normal tissue is heterozygous for a pair of alleles (Fig. 6.8). This procedure is referred to as loss-of-heterozygosity analysis. If loss of an allele is found consistently in a set of tumours of similar pathology, it provides evidence for chromosomal regions worth further examination in the search for tumour-suppressor genes (Table 6.4).

The data in Table 6.4, although incomplete, suggest that quite large numbers of genes must be involved in tumorigenesis. Several different cancer genes may be involved in the same tumour, a conclusion already reached from analysis of Wilms' tumour. The same genes may be lost or mutated in different types of cancer, a conclusion already observed in the discussion of the involvement of the RB gene in both retinoblastoma and osteosarcoma. It is also possible that there may be an ordered or sequential loss of tumour-suppressor genes as a cell progresses from predisposed to overtly cancerous. Finally, several of the chromosomal regions outlined in Table 6.4 also harbour oncogenes. Thus, loss-of-heterozygosity analysis cannot necessarily be equated with loss of tumour-suppressor genes.

THE p53 GENE

Unlike most other cancer genes, the p53 gene was first identified through its protein product, a nuclear phosphoprotein of 53 000 apparent molecular weight and found at high levels in mouse 3T3 cells transformed by a DNA tumour virus. Purification of the p53 protein enabled the controlling gene to be cloned and localized to the short arm of chromosome 17, a region that has been implicated in a number of different types of cancer (Table 6.4). Transfection experiments using p53 cDNA clones from normal mouse liver produced immortalized cell lines (see Fig. 6.3) and it thus seemed probable that p53 was another oncogene. However, it subsequently turned out that the cDNA clones in the transfection experiments had sustained a mutation during the cloning process, and that normal p53 genes had no oncogenic action.

It now seems that p53 should be seen as a tumour-suppressor gene, but one whose action throws further light on the complexities of tumour formation. Mutations in p53 are the most common genomic alterations found in human tumours, and have been observed in a wide variety of sporadic colorectal carcinomas, carcinomas of lung

Chromosomes 17

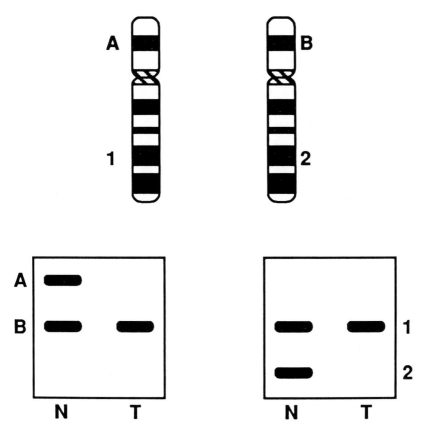

Fig. 6.8. Loss-of-heterozygosity analysis for two regions of chromosome 17 in breast cancer. The individual is heterozygous for markers A and B on the short arm and for markers 1 and 2 on the long arm of chromosome 17. Southern blot analysis of DNA from normal (N) and tumour (T) tissue shows that chromosomes 17 in the tumour tissue have lost allele A from the short arm and allele 2 from the long arm.

Table 6.4. *Chromosomal regions implicated in human cancers through loss-of-heterozygosity analysis*

Chromosomal region	Type of cancer
1p	Melanoma, neuroblastoma, ductal cell breast carcinoma, multiple endocrine neoplasia type 2, medullary thyroid carcinoma, phaeochromocytoma
1q	Breast cancer
3p	Small cell lung cancer, renal cell carcinoma, cervical carcinoma, von Hippel–Lindau disease, testicular cancer, breast cancer
5q	Colorectal carcinoma, FAP, Gardner syndrome
11p	Wilms' tumour, WAGR, Beckwith–Wiedemann syndrome, rhabdomyosarcoma, breast carcinoma, hepatoblastoma, transitional cell bladder carcinoma, adrenocortical carcinoma, testicular cancer
11q	Multiple endocrine neoplasia type 1
13q	Retinoblastoma, osteosarcoma, small cell lung cancer, ductal cell breast cancer, stomach cancer
17p	Small cell lung cancer, colorectal carcinoma, breast cancer, osteosarcoma
17q	Breast cancer
18q	Colorectal carcinoma, breast cancer
22q	Meningioma, acoustic neuroma, phaeochromocytoma, colorectal carcinoma

Source: Adapted from Sager (1989).

and breast, osteosarcomas, soft tissue sarcomas, brain tumours and leukaemias. In many of these tumours, homozygous loss of p53 genes and the absence of p53 mRNA suggested a model akin to that found in retinoblastoma. However, in other tumours and particularly in colorectal carcinomas, a mutant p53 allele on one chromosome was associated with a normal p53 allele on the homologous chromosome. Here was an example of a tumour-suppressor gene acting in a dominant–negative or gain-of-function fashion: in other words mutation in a single copy of the gene could promote tumour formation.

Although the full story of p53 action is far from complete, it is beginning to be possible to formulate a model for its involvement in cell proliferation. The normal product of the p53 gene is a homodimeric protein capable of binding DNA, and with presumed growth-regulating properties. It is expressed in a wide variety of cells, but at low levels because it is degraded rapidly by cellular proteases. Mutation in a p53 gene produces a mutant protein that can form a heterodimeric complex with the product of the normal p53 gene (Fig. 6.9). This leads to two possible mechanisms for cell proliferation. The

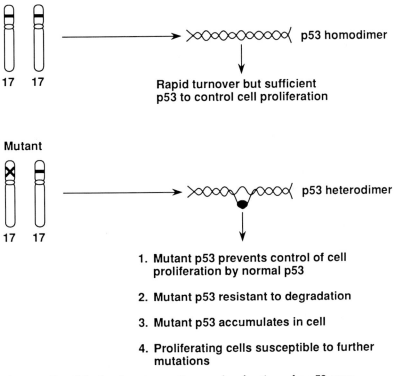

Fig. 6.9. Possible dominant–negative mode of action of a p53 gene. Mutation in a single copy of a p53 gene on chromosome 17 (**X**) leads to the formation of heterodimeric p53 protein, with one or more of the consequences shown.

159

Table 6.5. *Cancers in Li–Fraumeni syndrome families*

Type of cancer	% of individuals with this as first cancer by age 60
Breast carcinoma	25
Soft tissue carcinoma	12
Brain tumour	12
Osteosarcoma	6
Leukaemia	6
Adrenocortical carcinoma	1

Source: From Malkin et al. (1990).

mutant p53 protein may prevent the normal p53 protein from exerting its growth-suppressing function, the dominant–negative effect already referred to. Alternatively, or perhaps additionally, the mutant p53 protein might be resistant to proteolytic degradation. This would explain the high levels of mutant p53 protein observed in many tumour cells. Both mechanisms would confer growth advantage on cells, which, in proliferating, would become susceptible to further somatic mutations either in the normal copy of the p53 gene or in other tumour-suppressor genes or proto-oncogenes.

This view is reinforced by recent findings in a rare genetic disorder known as the Li–Fraumeni syndrome. The disorder is inherited as an autosomal dominant and affected individuals are highly susceptible to early development of a range of unrelated tumours (Table 6.5), of which breast cancer is the most common. In these families a mutant p53 gene is inherited in the germ line, with a striking positional clustering of point mutations between codons 245 and 258 of the gene. However, although affected individuals have inherited a mutant gene, which in sporadic tumours may act in dominant fashion, they do not usually succumb to overt cancer for at least 30 years. It is possible that the specific p53 mutations found in Li–Fraumeni families are in themselves weak tumour initiators but, because of their ubiquitous cellular distribution, they render an overt cancer a highly probable event in the long run. It is also possible that a mutation in the p53 gene in early life (inherited or germ line) is less damaging to the cell than a mutation in p53 arising after other somatic genome mutations.

In the Li–Fraumeni syndrome, p53 mutations occur in a limited area of the gene (codons 245 to 258), representing an evolutionarily conserved domain of the p53 protein. Other p53 mutations are more widely dispersed between codons 130 and 290 (out of 393), although there are hotspots at codons 175, 248 and 273 (Figure 6.10). One striking example of positional clustering is in a type of liver cancer found in both black South African and Chinese patients, where tumours contain G→T mutations in codon 249. Both aflatoxin and hepatitis B virus have been implicated in the aetiology of these cancers. Although the mutation occurs in the same domain of the p53 protein found in Li–Fraumeni patients, the effect appears to be more powerful, with a gain-of-function mechanism.

FAMILIAL ADENOMATOUS POLYPOSIS (FAP)

FAP is one of the more common autosomal dominant diseases with cancer predisposition, occurring at a frequency of 1 in 5000 to 1 in 10 000. It is characterized by the development during adolescence of thousands of polyps throughout the colon, and these progress, almost inevitably, to cancer unless the large bowel is removed surgically. The penetrance of the gene responsible for FAP is high, so that first-degree relatives of affected individuals have a 50% risk and often undergo frequent sigmoidoscopies in the search for malignant transformation. Congenital hypertrophy of the retinal pigment epithelium (CHRPE) is found in many gene carriers, but is associated with too many false positives and false negatives to be a reliable alternative screening test. In the related condition, Gardner syndrome, there are additional extra-colonic lesions in the form of multiple osteomas, epidermoid cysts and desmoid tumours.

In 1987 the gene for FAP was mapped to the long arm of chromo-

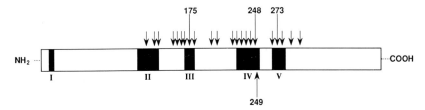

Fig. 6.10. Representation of the p53 protein with five evolutionarily conserved domains (I–V). Short arrows indicate regions in which mutations have been observed, and longer arrows indicate mutational hotspots. The specific mutation in codon 249 found in liver cancer is indicated below.

some 5 by cytogenetic and linkage analysis. Subsequent studies suggested that Gardner syndrome and FAP were allelic variants at the same locus. Saturation of the 5q21 region with DNA probes provided markers bracketing the locus and permitting presymptomatic detection of FAP gene carriers by indirect tracking. This also set the stage for cloning of the gene responsible. The first candidate gene to be isolated, referred to as MCC (mutated in colonic cancer), showed mutations in about 15% of sporadic carcinomas but not in the germ line of individuals with FAP. Further search of the 5q21 region revealed another expressed gene in which mutations occurred not only in sporadic colon tumours but also in the germ line of both FAP and Gardner syndrome patients. There seems little doubt that this gene (APC, adenomatous polyposis coli) is the inherited component of both FAP and Gardner syndrome.

The close proximity of two genes, MCC and APC, on the long arm of chromosome 5, and both implicated in colon cancers, raises a number of questions about function. There are as yet few clues to the nature of the encoded products, except that there are similarities to proteins regulating the cell-signalling pathways mediated by G proteins. It would appear that the APC gene is a tumour-suppressor; inactivation or point mutation of this gene is likely to lead to proliferation of the colonic mucosa, but actual polyp formation probably requires a second hit in the same gene, or in MCC or in other genes. There is thus a degree of similarity to retinoblastoma, with predisposition to malignancy being inherited in dominant fashion. However, in a fashion more akin to the situations seen in Wilms' and Li–Fraumeni patients, the second mutation is more likely to involve other genes.

ONCOGENES AND TUMOUR-SUPPRESSOR GENES

In the preceding sections a distinction was made between oncogenes and tumour-suppressor genes. In the classical view, normal cellular oncogenes (proto-oncogenes) are activated by a mutational event and provide the accelerator for cell proliferation. In contrast, tumour-suppressor genes are an inbuilt braking system against runaway cell proliferation, and in the model system of retinoblastoma, genes on a homologous pair of chromosomes must be inactivated or deleted before the brakes are released. However, data from both Wilms' tumour and the p53 gene have already shown that this simple model is inadequate. Mutation or deletion of a single copy of these tumour-suppressor genes, in association with other unknown changes in the genome, may be sufficient to produce a tumour. This raises a number of questions. Are tumour-suppressor genes simple braking systems or do they have more complicated roles in the cellular machinery? Is there any direct cellular connection between oncogenes and tumour-suppressor genes? Can the term anti-oncogene be used with any confidence in describing a tumour-suppressor gene?

The first suggestion of a connection between an oncogene and a tumour-suppressor gene came from the study of a group of DNA tumour viruses. In contrast to the oncogenes of retroviruses, which have been transduced from host cells, the oncogenes of DNA viruses have no direct host-cell counterpart. Whereas the protein products of retroviral oncogenes are largely irrelevant to the life cycle of the virus, the protein products of DNA viral oncogenes are intimately related to the life cycle of the virus and serve to create a suitable cellular environment for viral propagation. In the course of this parasitic activity, the oncogene product may occasionally transform the host cell into a malignant phenotype. There is now evidence that at least one mechanism for transformation may involve interaction with products of host tumour-suppressor genes.

The large T-antigen of simian virus 40 (SV40) is important both in viral replication and in host-cell transformation. It has been found that large T-antigen binds tightly and specifically both to the product of the retinoblastoma (RB) locus and to p53 proteins, though different domains of the T-antigen are involved. Similarly, the E1A and E1B transforming proteins of adenoviruses, and the E6 and E7 proteins of human papilloma virus, are found in cellular extracts, in complexes with the RB and p53 proteins. Thus, at least in the case of DNA tumour viruses, there is suggestive evidence of an interaction between an oncogene product and a tumour-suppressor gene product. It is quite possible that one of the modes of action of oncogenes may be in removing some of the braking effects of tumour-suppressor genes.

An even more intriguing connection between oncogenes and tumour-suppressor genes has surfaced following the cloning of the gene responsible for type 1 (Von Recklinghausen) neurofibromatosis (NF-1). The NF-1 gene has a number of unusual features, not least of which is the presence of three smaller genes within a large intron of NF-1 that are transcribed in the direction opposite to that of the NF-1 gene. However, the most exciting property of the NF-1 gene is that it encodes a protein with strong sequence homology to mammalian GTPase-activating proteins (GAPs) as well as to their yeast equivalents. GAPs are cytosolic proteins that catalyse the conversion of the active GTP-bound $p21^{ras}$ proteins to the inactive GDP-bound form. Although the exact function of GAPs is unknown, they are obviously important in down-regulating the activity of the products of *ras* oncogenes. It is therefore possible that the product of the NF-1 tumour-suppressor gene is also involved in the control of the action of *ras* oncogenes. This is the first example of a probable linkup between a tumour-suppressor gene and a cellular oncogene.

TOWARDS A MOLECULAR MODEL FOR CARCINOGENESIS

In 1975, Richard Peto and colleagues, in summarizing epidemiological evidence for multistage processes underlying the generation of the more common age-dependent human cancers, suggested that between four and six independent, rate-limiting steps were necessary. At the time this might have seemed a large number. Following the discovery of oncogenes and tumour-suppressor genes, it is probably on the conservative side. Values ranging from 8 to 15 somatic hits are now cited. As Bernard Weinstein said (quoted by Marx, 1989) 'a few years ago the question was whether there are genetic changes in cancer cells. Now you find a huge number of DNA changes. In cancer the genome is shot to hell.'

This may seem something of a counsel of despair, with the implication that a large number of random somatic changes contribute to the development of the cancer cell. In all probability it is a somewhat exaggerated statement, and in at least some cancers the number and sequence of mutational events is beginning to emerge. One important group are the colorectal carcinomas, among the most common malignancies in humans. Abundant clinical and histopathological data suggest that most of these arise from benign adenomatous polyps that proceed through a series of steps to full malignancy. Tumours at various stages of development from small adenomas to large metastatic carcinomas can be removed surgically and the range of somatic changes correlated with the histopathological stage. In a majority of these tumours, whether sporadic or the result of inheritance of FAP or Gardner syndrome, allele loss in the 5q region (this, of course includes allele inactivation through point mutation or other mechanisms) seems to be the precipitating event.

A possible model for colorectal carcinoma, proposed by Fearon and Vogelstein, is shown in Fig. 6.11. In patients with FAP, a mutation in the APC gene is the inherited predisposing event. In sporadic colorectal cancers, an early somatic mutation may occur in APC, or in MCC, or in other 5q genes. This gives rise to widespread hyperproliferation of the colonic epithelium and the formation of an early

164

adenoma. In early adenomatous cells the genomic DNA loses methyl groups by an as yet unknown mechanism, and this may contribute to subsequent chromosome changes during mitosis. One of these changes probably involves activation of the K-*ras* proto-oncogene, since K-*ras* gene mutations are observed in about 50% of adenomas greater than 1 cm in size but in less than 10% of smaller adenomas.

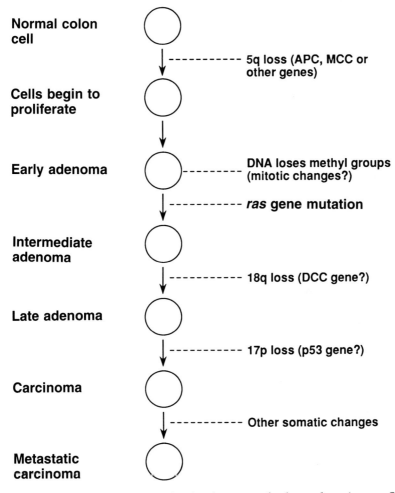

Fig. 6.11. A possible scheme for development of colorectal carcinoma. See the text for details. Adapted from Fearon and Vogelstein (1990). Copyright © Cell Press.

Clonal expansion of the early adenoma to an intermediate adenoma is followed by allele loss on chromosomes 18q and 17p. The latter is the site of the p53 tumour-suppressor gene described earlier. The 18q region harbours another putative tumour-suppressor gene called DCC (deleted in colorectal carcinoma), whose protein product is homologous to a range of cell-surface adhesion molecules. Evidence that loss of DCC precedes that of p53 is provided by the finding that colorectal carcinomas displaying deletions in region 17p are more aggressive than those with no loss of 17p alleles.

It must be pointed out that the model presented in Fig. 6.11 is still speculative. Although the order of events is likely it is not invariant, and adenomas have been observed in which loss of 17p preceded that of 5q and 18q, or where loss of 18q preceded a *ras* mutation. Fearon and Vogelstein emphasize that it is the accumulation rather than the order of events that is important. They point out that in more than 90% of the colorectal carcinomas they examined there was accumulation of more than two of the mutations shown in Fig. 6.11, whereas for early adenomas the figure was only 7%. Once a carcinoma has formed, the tumour may continue to grow and to metastasize, perhaps involving further as-yet uncharacterized mutations.

To what extent is it possible to generalize from a colorectal carcinoma model in Fig. 6.11 to other common cancers? It is clearly a preliminary scheme, likely to be adapted and modified. Other genes may be more important in other cancers. In small cell lung cancer, for example, the retinoblastoma gene is deleted or defective in most cases, while there is also loss of heterozygosity on chromosome 3p. Allele loss at 17p (presumably the p53 gene) is shared with colorectal cancer. In primary breast tumours there are reports of multiple chromosomal region losses; 1p, 1q, 3p, 11p, 13q, 17p, 17q and 18q (Table 6.4). A gene for inherited susceptibility to breast cancer has been mapped by linkage analysis to 17q21. Thus, although the Fearon and Vogelstein model may be only a first step towards a molecular model for carcinogenesis, it does provide an important testable hypothesis.

SUGGESTED READING

Fearon, E. R. and Vogelstein, B. (1990). A genetic model for colorectal tumorigenesis. *Cell* **61**: 759–767.

Friend, S. H., Dryja, T. P. and Weinberg, R. A. (1988). Oncogenes and tumour-suppressing genes. *Science* **318**: 618–622.

Hollstein, M., Sidransky, D., Vogelstein, B. and Harris, C. C. (1991). p53 mutations in human cancers. *Science* **253**: 50–53.

Hunter, T. (1985). The proteins of oncogenes. *Scientific American* **62**: 60–68.

Knudson, A. G. (1986). Genetics of human cancer. *Annual Review of Genetics* **20**: 231–246.

Linder D. and Gartler, S. M. (1965). Glucose-6-phosphate dehydrogenase mosaicism: utilization as a cell marker in uterine leiomyomas. *Science* **150**: 67–69.

Malkin, D., Li, F. P., Strong, L. C., Fraumeni, J. F. Jr, Nelson, C. E., Kim, D. H., *et al.* (1990). Germline p53 mutations in a familial syndrome of breast cancer, sarcomas and other neoplasms. *Science* **250**: 1233–1238.

Marshall, C. J. (1989). Oncogenes and cell proliferation: an overview. In Glover, D. M. and Hames, B. D. (Editors) *Oncogenes*, pp. 1–22, IRL Press, Oxford.

Marx, J. (1989). Many gene changes found in cancer. *Science* **246**: 1386–1388.

Mitchell, C. D. (1991). Recessive oncogenes, anti-oncogenes and tumour suppression. *British Medical Bulletin* **47**: 136–156.

Peto, R., Roe, F. J. C., Lee, P. N., Levy, L. and Clack, J. (1975). Cancer and ageing in mice and man. *British Journal of Cancer* **32**: 411–426.

Ponder, B. A. J. (1990). Inherited predisposition to cancer. *Trends in Genetics* **6**: 213–218.

Sager, R. L. (1989). Tumour-suppressor genes: the puzzle and the promise. *Science* **246**: 1406–1411.

Smith, P. J. (1991). Carcinogenesis: molecular defences against carcinogens. *British Medical Bulletin* **47**: 3–20.

Soloman, E., Borrow, J. and Goddard, A. D. (1991). Chromosome aberrations and cancer. *Science* **254**: 1153–1160.

Stanbridge, E. J. (1990). Identifying tumour suppressor genes in human colorectal cancer. *Science* **247**: 12–13.

Stanbridge, E. J. and Nowell, P. C. (1990). Origins of human cancer revisited. *Cell* **63**: 867–874.

Steel, C. M. (1989). Oncogenes and anti-oncogenes in human cancer. *Proceedings of the Royal College of Physicians, Edinburgh* **19**: 413–430.

Weinberg, R. A. (1991). Tumour suppressor genes. *Science* **254**: 1138–1145.

Xu, G., O'Connell, P., Viskochil, D., Cawthon, R., Robertson, M., Culver, M., *et al.* (1990). The neurofibromatosis type 1 gene encodes a protein related to GAP. *Cell* **62**: 599–608.

7 MOLECULAR CYTOGENETICS

Chromosomes were first recognized in the nineteenth century. Their ability to take up stains (Greek: chromos, colour; soma, body) implies a cytological mode of investigation, and the science of cytogenetics uses the microscope as the primary tool. The most widely used technique, Giemsa or G-banding, permits visualization of chromosome bands representing about 4000 to 5000 kb of genomic DNA. Although arresting dividing cells in prometaphase can increase the resolution by a factor of two, 2000 kb is still much larger than the size of even moderate genes (for example, the cystic fibrosis gene is 250 kb; the factor VIII gene is 180 kb). A visible chromosome band could contain quite a large number of smaller genes.

The advent of molecular genetic technology permits the structure and segregation of chromosomes to be studied by a completely new range of procedures that can be fruitfully combined with the use of the light microscope. These techniques, which may be loosely referred to as molecular cytogenetic, have contributed enormously to the understanding of the structure of chromosomes and their behaviour during meiosis and mitosis, as well as to delineating cytogenetic abnormalities that cannot be seen under the microscope. Some coverage of this topic has already been presented in Chapter 6, where loss-of-heterozygosity analysis in detecting cancer genes was reviewed (see p. 156). Other significant aspects of molecular cytogenetics are discussed below.

GENE MAPPING
Every few years, since 1973, an international human gene mapping workshop is held that leads to the publication of an updated map of gene assignments to the 23 human chromosomes. HGM11, held in 1991, produced a map with 2086 confirmed autosomal and 221 confirmed X-linked assignments. This exercise, which began as something of an academic sideshow, is now taken very seriously and is an

integral part of a larger programme to map and sequence the entire human genome. But while there may be arguments about the value of mapping regions of the genome that have no apparent function, there is no doubt about the practical benefits of locating specific genes (especially those responsible for particular diseases) at precise sites on their respective chromosomes. Not only has this made possible prenatal diagnosis and carrier detection of a variety of Mendelian disorders (Chapter 5), but gene mapping is becoming an important first step in the cloning of genes known only through their gross phenotypic effects. This procedure, known as reverse genetics or positional cloning, enables the function of a gene to be deduced from analysis of homologies to other known genes.

Before 1950 gene mapping was restricted largely to the X chromosome, where characteristic patterns of inheritance allowed localizations to be made by pedigree inspection. In the last 40 years a number of laboratory methods have emerged that allow genes to be assigned not only to particular chromosomes but to quite precise bands and subbands within chromosomal regions. These techniques are greatly assisted by linkage analysis (Chapter 5), which allows two or more genes to be placed in the same linkage group. If one of the genes in the group already has a chromosomal assignment then all the other genes in the linkage group may be assigned to the same chromosomal region. But if this is not the case, at least one of the genes in the group will need a physical assignment to a chromosome before the linkage group can be regarded as mapped.

Methods for chromosomal assignment of genes are becoming remarkably sophisticated. Historically, two procedures have dominated the elaboration of the human map – somatic-cell hybridization and in situ hybridization – and these are discussed below.

IN SITU HYBRIDIZATION
The most direct method of localizing a cloned DNA sequence (whether representing a functional gene or an anonymous DNA segment) to a specific chromosome is by in situ hybridization. It depends on the fact that the cloned sequence (referred to as the probe), when rendered single-stranded by heating, will anneal to its complementary sequence in a denatured chromosome. The probe is first labelled with either a radioactive or a fluorescent tag and then applied to a spread of denatured metaphase chromosomes, which will still retain their characteristic configurations. After removal of excess labelled probe, the position of the maximum signal is identified on a specific chromosome.

169

For many years, labelling of probes with tritium has been a standard method for in situ hybridization. After completion of hybridization and washing, slides are dipped in a photographic emulsion and then stored for various periods of time. Disintegrations of the radioactive tritium produce silver grains in the emulsion, which can be scored against regions of specific chromosomes. There is inevitably a certain amount of background silver grain production, and it is normal practice to examine many chromosome spreads and thus to build up a composite picture of the most likely region of hybridization. A typical histogram, constructed in this way, is shown in Fig. 7.1. Disadvantages of the method are: (a) the scatter of disintegrations around the region of hybridization may reduce the precision of localization; (b) long periods of time may be necessary for the acquisition of significant numbers of silver grains; and (c) high background levels of silver grains.

Non-isotopic labelling of probes with fluorochromes is now beginning to replace tritium labelling for in situ hybridization. After hybridization, the signal is visualized directly either by fluorescent microscopy or by laser-scanning confocal microscopy. There is no scattering of signal, no need for the laborious construction of histograms, and the whole process is complete in a matter of days (Fig. 7.2).

A further advantage of fluorescence labelling for in situ hybridization is that more than one probe may be used simultaneously, each labelled with a different fluorochrome. When such two-colour or multi-colour fluorescence is applied to prometaphase or interphase chromosomes (which are greatly extended compared to metaphase chromosomes), the relative positions of the probes can be deduced. Thus, not only are genes mapped to specific chromosomal regions, but the order of quite closely spaced genes (as little as 50 kb apart) along the chromosome may be established with some precision. Hybridization of multiple probes with differently coloured fluorescent tags is referred to as chromosome painting.

SOMATIC CELL HYBRIDIZATION

When human cell lines are fused to mouse cell lines by the use of viruses or chemical agents, the resulting interspecific hybrid initially contains a double chromosome complement. As the hybrid is passaged it begins preferentially to shed human chromosomes in a random fashion. Eventually the hybrid becomes relatively stable and

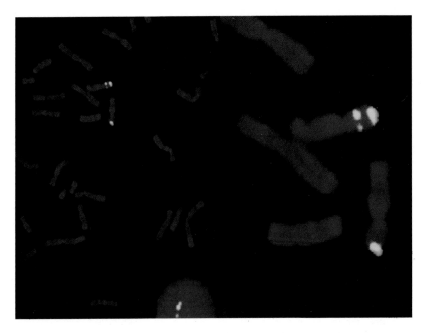

Fig. 7.2. In situ hybridization with fluorescently tagged markers. A set of metaphase chromosomes is shown on the left, and higher-power resolution of five chromosomes on the right. Two fluorescently tagged probes have been used. One detects the insulin gene at the tip of chromosome 11p, the other the Wilms' tumour gene at 11p13 (yellow fluorescence). Note that the Wilms' tumour gene has been deleted on one of the chromosomes 11 (see Chapter 6). Courtesy of Dr Judy Fantes.

Facing p.170

will grow for a number of cycles with a fixed chromosome complement. It is not possible to predict which human chromosomes will be
lost and which will be retained. It is possible, however, to examine
the hybrid cytogenetically and to ascertain which human chromosomes are present. If several such hybrid lines are created, they pro-

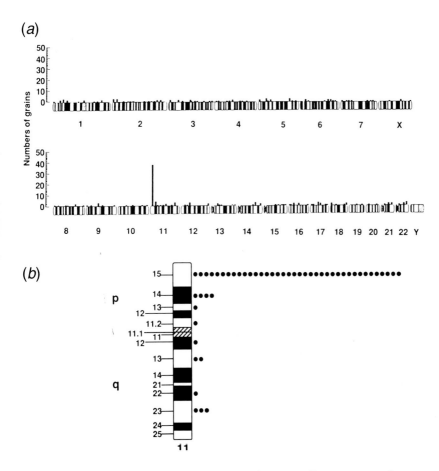

Fig. 7.1. Regional localization of the acid sphingomyelinase gene to the
short arm of chromosome 11 by in situ hybridization. (*a*)
Distribution of sites of hybridization among the 23 human
chromosomes. (*b*) Autoradiographic grains are concentrated at
11p15. From Pereira *et al.* (*Genomics* **9**: 222; 1991).

vide a panel of cells that differ in their human chromosome complements (Fig. 7.3).

Panels of somatic cell hybrids may be used in two different ways to map human genes. If a human gene has an expressed protein product that differs in physical characteristics from the corresponding mouse protein product, the human protein product may be searched for in homogenates of the different lines in the panel. Starch gel electrophoresis and specific staining of enzymes or the use of antibodies are standard methods of search. Lines that are positive for the human

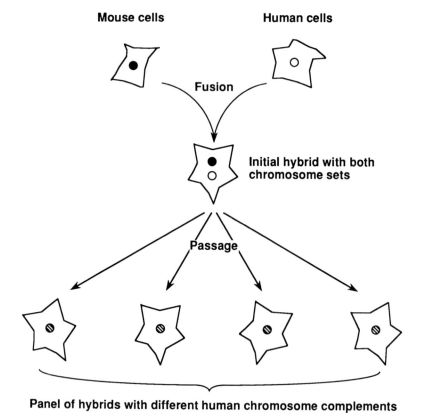

Panel of hybrids with different human chromosome complements

Fig. 7.3. Creation of a panel of somatic cell hybrids with different complements of human chromosomes.

172

protein must contain the controlling human gene, and examination of
the human chromosomes in the line will narrow the gene localization
usually to only a few chromosomes. By inspection of the whole panel
of lines, it is normally possible to construct a grid (Fig. 7.4) in which
only one human chromosome correlates invariably with the specific
gene product.

A more powerful method of using somatic cell hybrids is to
hybridize the lines in the panel to a radiolabelled copy of a probe
representing the gene of interest. The hybrid cells are first digested
with a restriction endonuclease that cuts the DNA into suitably sized
fragments, and the fragments then separated by agarose electrophoresis and blotted by conventional Southern methodology. Since
the human chromosome complement of the different lines in the
panel will be known in advance, those that show positive or negative
signals on hybridization with a radiolabelled probe can be used to
construct a grid similar to that shown in Fig. 7.4. The advantage of
this method is that it can be used to map human genes that do not
express a protein product in the hybrid; indeed it can be used for any
DNA sequence complementary to a region on a human chromosome.

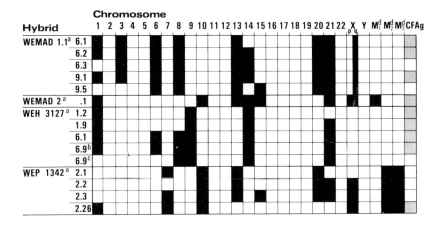

Fig. 7.4. The segregation of human chromosomes and a specific human
protein (CFAg) in subclones from a series of four independent
mouse–human hybrids. Note that the only chromosome to
correlate exactly with the presence of CFAg (shaded squares on
right) is chromosome 1. From van Heyningen *et al.* (*Nature
(London)* **315:** 513; 1985).

OTHER METHODS

In situ hybridization and somatic cell hybrids, particularly when combined with linkage analysis, are powerful tools for mapping genes that show Mendelian modes of segregation. However, they are by no means the only procedures available to the molecular geneticist. The importance of chromosomal aberrations in delineating regions of possible significance for genes, of both known and unknown function, is discussed later in this chapter. Loss-of-heterozygosity analysis in pinpointing putative tumour-suppressor genes was outlined in Chapter 6.

Another type of gene mapping procedure is referred to as dosage analysis. It depends on the fact that the level of gene product in a cell is generally related to the number of intact alleles at an autosomal locus. If an individual is a heterozygote for a particular genetic disorder because of a gene deletion, he or she will produce only about 50% of the gene product. In some cases it is possible to correlate heterozygous expression of the gene product with cytogenetic evidence for the chromosomal region deleted. The same principle may be applied to chromosomal duplications, where the level of gene product is increased. Examples of gene dosage analysis are shown in Fig. 7.5.

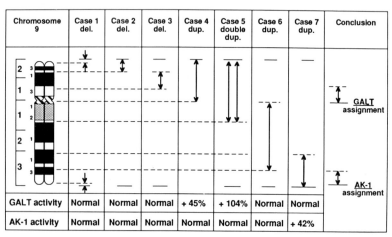

Fig. 7.5. Use of gene dosage to localize the enzymes galactose-1-phosphate uridyltransferase (GALT) and adenylate kinase 1 (AK-1) to chromosome 9. Enzyme activity is correlated with different deletion (del.) and duplication (dup.) aberrations. From Connor and Ferguson-Smith (1988) *Essential Medical Genetics*, 2nd Edition, Blackwell Scientific, Oxford.

THE HUMAN GENE MAP

The status of the human gene map changes almost by the week and is now quite complex. An example of a single chromosome is shown in Fig. 7.6. It includes cloned genes whose functions and positions are known with some certainty as well as uncloned genes known only by gross phenotypic effects. In addition, a very large number of anonymous DNA segments have been mapped to specific regions of all the human chromosomes. These are not shown in Fig. 7.6.

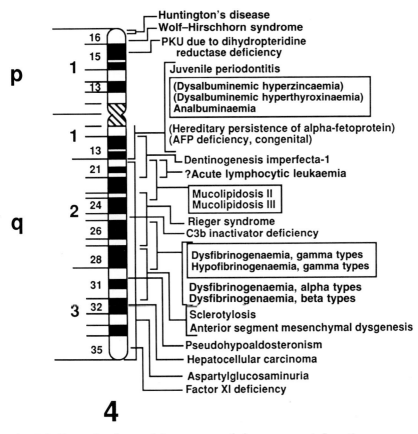

Fig. 7.6. Example of a partial gene map of chromosome 4. Locations are limited to genes responsible for a specific disorder.

X-CHROMOSOME INACTIVATION

In Chapter 2 (see p. 13) it was pointed out that in female somatic cells one of the two X chromosomes is randomly inactivated early in embryogenesis. In this way female cells achieve dosage equivalence with male cells, which have only a single X chromosome. The inactive X becomes heterochromatic and can be seen in the nucleus as a dark-staining mass known as a Barr body. The drive to dosage equivalence is so strong that in X-chromosome aneuploidies, such as XXX or XXXY, two Barr bodies can be seen in the nucleus. In general, the number of Barr bodies is one less than the total number of X chromosomes in the cell. The inactive X chromosome replicates late in the cell cycle and is, for the most part, genetically silent. This means that most genes carried on an inactive X chromosome produce no protein product.

Once X inactivation has occurred, in the trophoblast at about day 12 and in the embryo proper by day 16, there is stable inheritance of the same inactivated X chromosome through subsequent mitotic divisions – an example of genomic imprinting (see p. 179). Inactivation occurs at random, with either paternally or maternally-derived X chromosomes becoming genetically silent. It is also extremely stable, and only in ageing cells is there evidence for a gradual reactivation and expression of genes from the silent X chromosome. This is remarkable given that in each mitotic division the inactivated X must decondense and uncoil to allow DNA replication.

It has gradually become apparent, however, that a physical picture of a pyknotic X chromosome from which no genes can be transcribed is inadequate. There are several genes on the extreme tip of the short arm of the X chromosome that escape inactivation. One of these is XG, which controls the X-linked blood group, Xg. Others are: the steroid sulphatase gene (STS), which encodes an enzyme whose deficiency is responsible for X-linked ichthyosis; GS1, which encodes a putative membrane protein; and KALIG-1, responsible for Kallman syndrome (Fig. 7.7). All these map to the pseudoautosomal region of the X chromosome, which pairs with the short arm of the Y chromosome during meiosis, and undergoes recombination. Another gene, MIC2, which encodes a cell-surface antigen, also maps to this region and likewise escapes inactivation. Unlike the Xg and steroid sulphatase genes, MIC2 has a functional homologous gene on the short arm of the Y chromosome. All these genes are localized in the terminal 5 to 7 Mb of the short arm in band Xp22.3.

The idea that genes on the X chromosome escape inactivation by virtue of their position at the extreme tip of the short arm can no longer be sustained. There is now a growing list of more proximally localized genes that escape inactivation, including two that map to the long arm. Fig. 7.7 shows a picture of genes escaping inactivation interspersed with genes known to be subject to inactivation. Inacti-

Genes known to be subject to X inactivation

Genes known to escape X inactivation

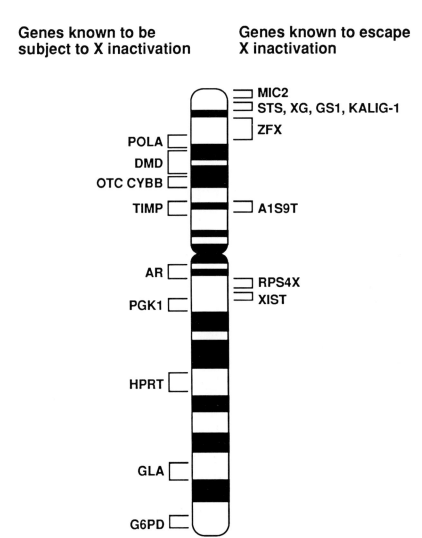

Fig. 7.7. Map of the human X chromosome showing genes escaping X inactivation and some of those subject to X inactivation.

vation appears to occur on a locus-by-locus basis, rather than by the physical shutting-down of whole chromosomal regions. Any model for the molecular mechanism of X inactivation must take into account this regional autonomy.

It has long been recognized that many X–autosome translocations, as well as some structurally abnormal chromosomes, remain active in cells while the normal X chromosome is preferentially inactivated. This suggests that there exists a controlling gene (or genes) responsible for shutting down the X chromosome on which it resides (known as acting in cis), which has been deleted or mutated in those

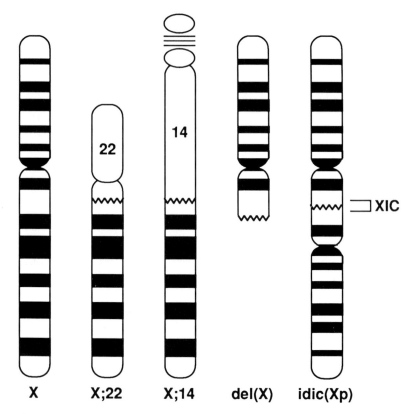

Fig. 7.8. Structurally abnormal X chromosome, each capable of being inactivated and therefore presumed to contain a common region harbouring the XIC gene. From Brown *et al.* (1991*b*). Reprinted by permission from *Nature (London)* **349:** 82–84. Copyright © 1991 Macmillan Magazines Ltd.

abnormal X chromosomes that always escape inactivation. Experiments in mice have identified an X-chromosome controlling element (Xce) in which mutations prevent inactivation. A similar element in humans (XIC, the X-inactivation centre) has been hypothesized to lie on the proximal long arm between Xq11.2 and Xq21.1.

Attempts to locate the X-inactivation centre have used the technique of SRO (smallest region of overlap), in which different abnormal X chromosomes are searched for a common region found on all inactivated chromosomes. As shown in Fig. 7.8 this has localized XIC to band 13 on the long arm, in a region bounded by XIST towards the telomere and DXS227 towards the centromere. DXS227 defines an anonymous probe whereas XIST produces RNA transcripts. There is now evidence that XIST may either be the X-inactivation centre itself, or else be closely involved in the inactivation process.

The most important function of the XIST gene is that it is transcribed from only inactivated X chromosomes. This was established by examining specific RNA transcripts from somatic cell hybrids in which either an inactivated or an activated X were the only human chromosomes present. The presence of stop codons in the sequenced exons of XIST suggests that it does not encode a protein product. In many ways this makes sense, for a protein product made on cytoplasmic ribosomes would have to return to the nucleus to perform its inactivating function. In contrast, an RNA molecule could act immediately on other loci on the X chromosome without needing to leave the cell nucleus.

A tentative model for X inactivation is presented in Fig. 7.9. The first step would be the blocking of the XIC on the active X chromosome by some unknown factor. Such blocked chromosomes would continue to express their entire complement of genes. The unblocked XIC on the homologous X chromosome would now be free to produce XIST RNA, which would spread the inactivation signal to those genes on the same chromosome (acting in cis), capable of receiving it. Most of the expressed genes on this (the inactivated) X chromosome would be shut down and genetically silent, the exceptions presumably being incapable of receiving an inactivation signal.

GENOMIC IMPRINTING

According to Mendelian principles, it should not be possible to distinguish the parental origin of identical homologous chromosomes in a zygote. Much of our understanding of the transmission of human genetic diseases is founded in the idea that the parental origin of a mutant gene is irrelevant to the expression of the phenotype. For

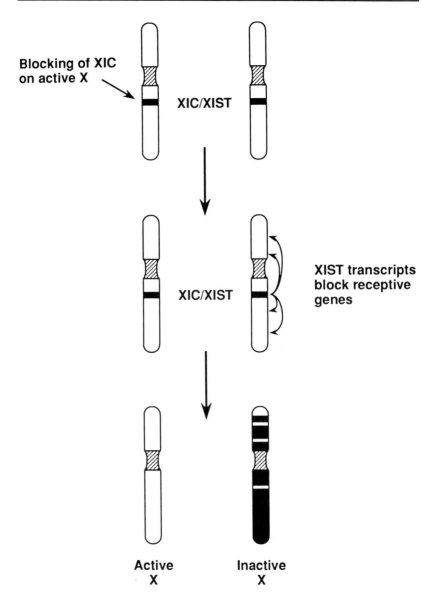

Fig. 7.9. A possible model for X inactivation. The initial step is blocking of XIC on one X chromosome by an unknown factor. XIC on the homologous X chromosome produces transcripts that act in cis to inactivate receptive genes. Most, but not all, of this X chromosome becomes inactive. The hatched region represents the centromere.

example, in dominantly inherited disorders, affected fathers and affected mothers each have a 50% chance of affected offspring, while in Down syndrome the extra chromosome 21 can come from either parent. However, there are some important exceptions to this fundamental principle. Whole chromosomes, specific chromosomal regions or even single genes may be marked in some mysterious way during germ-cell lineage and the consequent phenotype of the zygote then becomes dependent on the parental origin on the mutant gene or genes. This phenomenon is known as genomic imprinting or sometimes just imprinting. Evidence for imprinting in humans comes from a variety of sources: chromosome sets, individual chromosomes, chromosomal regions and the expression of specific genes.

CHROMOSOME SETS

Hydatidiform moles occur in about 1 in 1500 recognized pregnancies. The karyotype is usually 46,XX (rarely 46,XY), but in both cases there are two paternally derived sets of haploid chromosomes and no maternal contribution. Although the chromosome complement is normal, complete moles are characterized by widespread hyperplasia of the trophoblast and the absence of a fetus. The paternal, or androgenetic, origin of the genome is inadequate for the formation of a functional zygote. In contrast, ovarian teratomas (dermoid cysts) have two maternal sets of haploid chromosomes, indicating that a gynogenetic origin of the genome is also inadequate for the formation of a fetus.

In triploid fetuses there is an extra set of either paternal or maternal chromosomes. Survival to term is unusual and few triploids are born alive. When the additional chromosome complement is paternal, the placenta is usually large and cystic and often associated with a partial hydatidiform mole. When there are two maternal chromosome complements and one paternal, the placenta is normally underdeveloped. This supports the idea, derived from nuclear transplantation experiments in the mouse, that paternal genetic information plays a critical role in the growth and maintenance of the placenta and membranes (Table 7.1). However, these results give no information regarding which chromosome or chromosomal regions are involved.

INDIVIDUAL CHROMOSOMES

It is possible, in principle, for a child to receive two copies of a particular chromosome from one parent and no copy from the other parent – a phenomenon known as uniparental disomy. Establishing that this can occur in humans is difficult, and is largely dependent on

181

Table 7.1. *Abnormalities in chromosome sets*

Syndrome	Chromosome abnormality	Phenotype
Hydatidiform mole	Two paternal haploid sets	Hyperplasia of trophoblast, absent fetus
Ovarian teratoma	Two maternal haploid sets	Completely disorganised fetal tissues
Triploid fetus	Extra paternal haploid set	Large cystic placenta, embryo stunted/malformed
Triploid fetus	Extra maternal haploid set	Small fibrotic placenta, embryo underdeveloped

a chance observation followed by detailed analysis of the disomy with a range of molecular markers. However, in experimental animals, uniparental disomies can be engineered. Highly inbred strains of mice are a particularly valuable resource for this purpose. In the first place it can be assumed that homologous chromosomes carry identical sets of genes and thus the significance of the parental origin of the chromosome can be assessed without fear that effects are due to different genes. Secondly, homologies between mouse and human chromosomes are now well established, and a mouse chromosome showing an imprinting effect can often be matched to an equivalent human chromosome or chromosomal region.

One of the tools used in studies on mice was the creation of mouse lines in which one or more pairs of homologous chromosomes were fused (Fig. 7.10). During meiosis, such fused chromosomes will be unable to separate and will pass as a unit to the gamete, so that some gametes will have two copies of a specific chromosome and others none. Crossing of such mouse lines can, therefore, generate both types of uniparental disomy, one containing the fused pair of chromosomes from the mother and the other the fused pair from the father. Since the mice are highly inbred, the offspring should be identical. In fact, for certain chromosomes this is not the case. In particular, mouse chromosomes 2 and 11 have quite distinct and opposite effects. Mouse pups with two chromosomes 2 or 11 from the mother are small and hypoactive, while a paternal origin for these chromosomes leads to large size and hyperactivity. Several other mouse chromosomes and chromosomal segments also show evidence of imprinting.

The first clear example of a uniparental disomy in humans was reported in 1988. It involved a young girl with cystic fibrosis and short

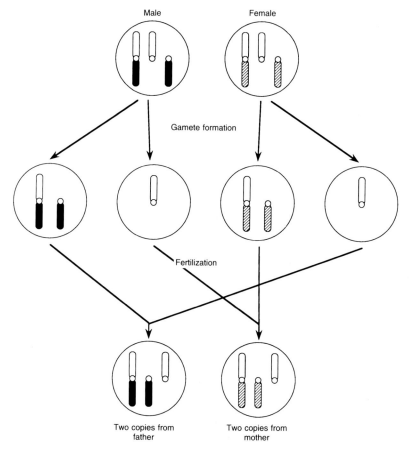

Fig. 7.10. The use of fused chromosomes to demonstrate imprinting effects in mice. In each of the male and female somatic cells (top) there has been fusion between non-homologous acrocentric chromosomes. The fused chromosomes pass intact to the gametes, and thus the zygote inheriting a fused chromosome will have either two paternal or two maternal copies of one chromosome.

183

stature who had inherited two copies of her mother's chromosome 7 and no chromosome 7 from the father. Another case, also involving cystic fibrosis and short stature, was discovered soon afterwards. In both cases non-paternity was essentially eliminated by detailed analysis of highly polymorphic markers. The DNA analysis of the second case is shown in Fig. 7.11. It can be seen that the child has a duplicated copy of one of the maternal chromosomes (isodisomy). How this has happened is not known. It is also not clear whether the short stature in the child is the consequence of the absence of a paternal chromosome 7 and therefore an example of imprinting, or whether it is the result of homozygosity for another gene (or genes)

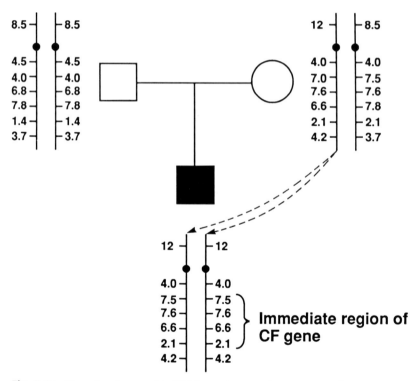

Fig. 7.11. Use of polymorphic DNA markers to demonstrate that an affected cystic fibrosis (CF) boy has inherited two copies of the same maternal chromosome 7 (uniparental isodisomy). Squares represent male individuals; circles represent females. Open symbols represent individuals of unaffected or undetermined status; the filled symbol represents the affected individual.

on chromosome 7. At least 22 genetic loci on human chromosome 7 have known homologies on mouse chromosomes; these include loci on mouse chromosomes 2 and 11, where maternal disomy has been shown to lead to small size at birth.

CHROMOSOMAL REGIONS

Probably the most clear-cut example of genomic imprinting in humans comes from the study of two clinically distinct but cyto-genetically indistinguishable disorders – the Angelman and Prader–Willi syndromes. In Angelman syndrome (Fig. 7.12*a*), also known as happy puppet syndrome, children have severe motor and intellectual retardation, ataxic gait, hypotonia and a facies with a large mandible, wide mouth and protruding tongue. Prader–Willi syndrome (Fig. 7.12*b*) is marked by neonatal hypotonia and failure to thrive, short stature, obesity and mild to moderate mental retardation. About half of each group of patients have a de novo deletion of part of the long arm of chromosome 15 that is either cytogenetically visible or detect-able by analysis of flanking DNA markers. The 15q11–q13 region affected appears to be the same in both syndromes.

Careful analysis of DNA polymorphisms has shown that in Angel-man syndrome the deletion arises on the maternally derived chromo-some 15, whereas in Prader–Willi syndrome it arises on the paternally derived chromosome 15. This is reinforced by the finding that a minority of cases of both syndromes may result from uniparental disomies, Angelman cases inheriting two paternal chromosomes 15 and Prader–Willi cases two maternal chromosomes 15. In both syn-dromes uniparental isodisomy (a single parental chromosome 15, which is duplicated) as well as uniparental heterodisomy (both chromosomes 15 from one parent) have been observed (Fig. 7.13). This suggests that Angelman syndrome is caused by the absence of a critical region of the maternal chromosome 15 and Prader–Willi by the absence of a critical region on the paternal chromosome 15. It is still not entirely clear that exactly the same chromosomal regions are involved in the two distinct syndromes, but the bulk of the evidence suggests that this is the case and that imprinting is responsible for the clinical differences.

It was pointed out in Chapter 6 that tumour-suppressor genes can be inactivated either by mutation at a specific genetic locus or by loss of a chromosomal region containing the gene. The latter event is often detected by analysis of DNA markers indicating loss of heterozy-gosity in tumour tissue. In principle, loss of heterozygosity could affect either the paternally derived or the maternally derived chromosome. There is now evidence that in some tumours preferential loss of one or other chromosome or chromosomal region occurs. In sporadic cases of Wilms' tumour and in sporadic rhabdomyosarcomas there is a bias towards loss of segments on the short arm of the maternal chromosome 11, and in sporadic osteosarcomas and retinoblastomas there is preferential loss of the maternal retinoblastoma gene on 13q. In contrast, in Beckwith–Wiedemann syndrome there is duplication of a paternally derived 11p15.5 region. One way of explaining this is to suggest the maternal tumour-suppressor alleles are repressed, relative to paternally derived alleles, by

(a)

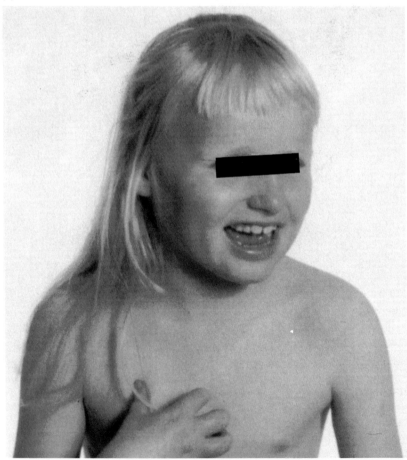

imprinting, and that mutation in the active paternal allele is sufficient to initiate cell proliferation and the type of cancerous growth that eventually eliminates the inactive maternal chromosome. However, this is an entirely speculative hypothesis, and may not stand the test of further experimental observations.

(b)

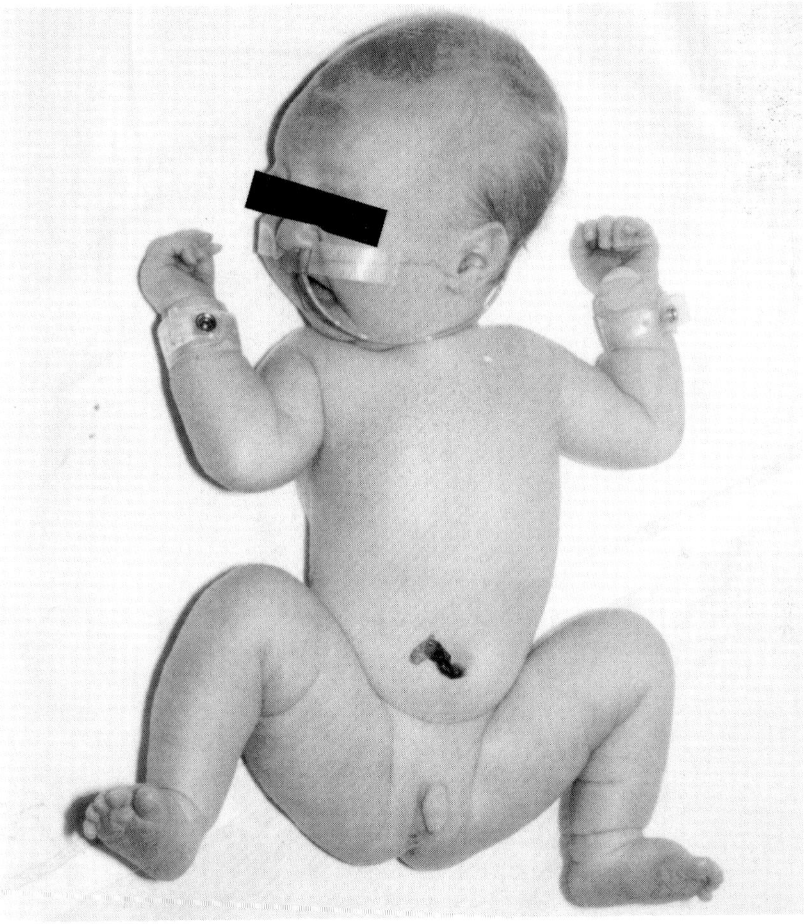

Fig. 7.12. A probable example of genomic imprinting. In both Angelman syndrome (*a*) and Prader–Willi syndrome (*b*) there may be a deletion of the 15q11–q13 region, in the former case involving a maternally derived chromosome and in the latter case a paternally derived chromosome. Courtesy of Dr John Tolmie.

Angelman syndrome   Prader-Willi syndrome

Deletion of 15qll-13

p m   p m

Parental isodisomy

p1 p1   m1 m1

Parental heterodisomy

 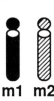

p1 p2   m1 m2

Fig. 7.13. Types of chromosome 15 found in Angelman and Prader–Willi syndromes. The top set illustrates deletions at 15q11–q13. The middle set shows parental isodisomies with a duplicated single paternal (Angelman) and a duplicated single maternal (Prader–Willi) chromosome 15. In the bottom set, the Angelman child has inherited both paternal chromosomes and the Prader–Willi child both maternal chromosomes. It is worth noting that the bottom set of chromosomes conferred no abnormality on the parents from whom they were derived.

SINGLE-GENE EFFECTS

The effect of imprinting on the expression of single genes is most easily studied in dominantly inherited disorders. Both males and females may transmit a mutant gene to affected offspring and the phenotypic consequences may then be correlated with paternal origins. An obvious confounding effect is the possibility of allelic heterogeneity at the locus under investigation, but this can be controlled by studying relatively rare genes in extended families where the assumption may be made that a single allele is involved. A more difficult confounding effect occurs with maternal transmission, since an affected female could, in theory, produce tissue factors that influence the expression of a mutant gene in her fetus while in the womb. This is a likely explanation for the severe childhood form of myotonic dystrophy, nearly always associated with maternal transmission of the mutant gene.

Huntington's disease shows wide variation in age of onset with a median at about age 45. A distinct subtype, juvenile Huntington's disease, with age of onset before 15 years, is characterized by mental retardation and rigidity rather than chorea. Most rigid cases inherit their mutant genes from their fathers, and this may well be an example of imprinting. A similar example is found in dominantly inherited spinocerebellar ataxia, where early onset tends to be associated with paternal transmission of the gene.

HOW DOES IMPRINTING OCCUR?

With the possible exceptions of the Prader–Willi and Angelman syndromes, the evidence for genomic imprinting in humans is still somewhat inconclusive. The belief that it is an important aspect of genetic transmission stems in a large part from experiments in other species, and in particular the mouse. It is now comparatively easy to create transgenic mice in which foreign genes are inserted into the germ line and where expression of the foreign gene (transgene) can be followed through successive generations. In up to a quarter of such transgenic strains, expression depends on the sex of the transmitting parent. In many cases paternally transmitted genes are expressed whereas maternally transmitted genes are not. More important, in paternally transmitted transgenes the DNA is undermethylated, whereas in maternally transmitted transgenes it is hypermethylated. This has lead to the suggestion that methylation is a key factor in regulating the expression of imprinted genes. This is not to say that methylation and imprinting are necessarily the same thing, but only that the correlation is sufficiently striking (at least in the mouse) to implicate DNA methylation as an important part of the imprinting process.

SEX DETERMINATION

The early embryonic gonad, although containing primordial germ cells from the fourth week, is essentially undifferentiated until the sixth or seventh week of development. In fact, the embryo is neither male nor female, since it contains both Müllerian and Wolffian ducts (Fig. 7.14). In the presence of a testis-determining factor (TDF), the gonad develops into a testis and elaborates two inducers. One is testosterone, which stimulates Wolffian duct proliferation and formation of the vas deferens. The other is the Müllerian inhibitory factor, which causes regression of the Müllerian duct. In the absence of TDF, the outer portion of the gonad develops into an ovary, the Wolffian duct regresses and the Müllerian duct develops into the upper portion of the vagina and into the uterus and the fallopian tubes.

According to this scheme, the embryonic gonad is inherently female unless influenced by TDF. Testis determining has thus become synonymous with male determining. Obviously, sex

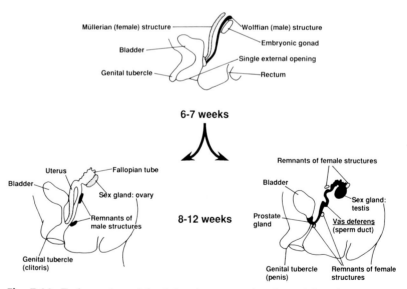

Fig. 7.14. Embryonic and fetal development of male and female sex organs. See the text for details.

determination is not as simple as this and there are examples of sex reversal that cannot be ascribed to TDF or its absence. However, there seems little doubt that a gene (or genes) encoding TDF is central to the differentiation of sexual characteristics during normal development. For this reason, considerable effort has been expended on cloning and identifying the gene controlling the male-determining factor.

As has happened many times in human genetics, the early clues to sex determination were provided by individuals with chromosome abnormalities. Soon after the normal human diploid chromosome complement was determined to be 46, it was discovered that phenotypically male Klinefelter syndrome patients were 46,XXY and that phenotypically female Turner syndrome patients were 45,X. The presence or absence of a Y chromosome, rather than the number of X chromosomes, was the critical factor. This was confirmed by the finding of 47,XXX and 48,XXXX females and 48,XXXY males.

Although the Y chromosome is one of the smallest of the human chromosomes, it still encompasses some 30 to 40 Mb of DNA, a large area to search for a putative TDF-controlling gene. The breakthrough was provided by the study of rare (1 in 20 000) XX males and even rarer (1 in 100 000) XY females. Careful cytogenetic analysis showed that in a proportion of XX males there had been a translocation of a portion of the short arm of the Y chromosome to the short arm of the X chromosome. In some XY females there had been a deletion of part of the short arm of the Y chromosome.

It made sense to assume that this translocated (XX males) or deleted (XY females) region of the Y chromosome contained the TDF gene. Mapping of the Y chromosome in XY females and of Y-chromosomal translocated segments in XX males, using batteries of DNA markers, shows the critical segment to consist of about 250 kb of DNA on the centromeric side of the pseudoautosomal region of the short arm of the Y chromosome (Fig. 7.15).

There is now excellent evidence that the gene for TDF has been cloned and characterized. The starting points for chromosome jumping and walking strategies were two highly informative sex-reversed patients, one an XX male and the other an XY female, and both of whom contained Y-chromosome sequences consisting of a narrow region just proximal to the pseudoautosomal pairing and exchange segment. The first candidate gene, called ZFY, was discounted on a number of grounds, one of which was the finding of a close homologue on the X chromosome. The second candidate gene, SRY (for sex-determining region of the Y), was a great deal more promising. It is Y specific in a range of eutherian mammals and absent from the human X chromosome. A homologous mouse gene, Sry, is expressed in gonadal tissue and this expression is limited to the period of development during which the testes begin to form. In XY females without deletions of the critical segment of the Y region shown in Fig. 7.15, de novo mutations in the SRY gene have been discovered. SRY encodes a protein with homologies to other DNA-binding proteins, and thus has the properties expected for a transcription regulator.

Final proof that SRY is indeed the master sex-determining gene depends on transgenic experiments in mice. Already it has been possible to introduce the Sry gene into XX mouse embryos and to observe the development of a male phenotype in some cases. Initial transduction of the human SRY gene into XX embryos was not successful, possibly for technical reasons. However, even if these experiments do eventually achieve the expected sex reversal, it must be remembered that sex determination can also be influenced by other genes not necessarily on the sex chromosomes. An obvious example is the 21-hydroxylase gene on chromosome 6, whose deficiency leads to one form of congenital adrenal hyperplasia and excessive virilization in females. Several other sexual ambiguity syndromes have been described that appear to be independent of abnormalities of the Y chromosome. Thus, if SRY is confirmed as the testis-determining factor gene, it will at best be primus inter pares in the complicated pathway of sex determination.

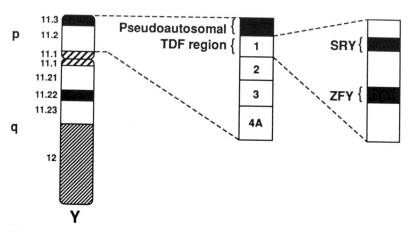

Fig. 7.15. The Y chromosome and successive exploded diagrams showing approximate positions of the SRY and ZFY genes in the area proximal to the pseudoautosomal region.

TELOMERES

When human chromosomes are viewed under the light microscope they are seen as discrete bodies with distinct ends – the telomeres. It has been known for some time that telomeres must have unusual and stabilizing properties. If a chromosome is broken in a cellular accident, the broken ends are 'sticky' and either fuse together again, or if there is another broken chromosome in the cell, cross-fuse to give a translocation chromosome. Normal telomeres do not behave in this way; they lack stickiness.

There is another peculiar property of telomeres, which follows from the nature of DNA replication. This was mentioned briefly in Chapter 3, and depends on the fact that DNA synthesis always occurs in a 5' to 3' direction. As a DNA duplex unwinds, replication of the 3' to 5' strand (the leading strand) occurs continuously in the direction of the advancing replication fork (Fig. 7.16). In contrast, replication of

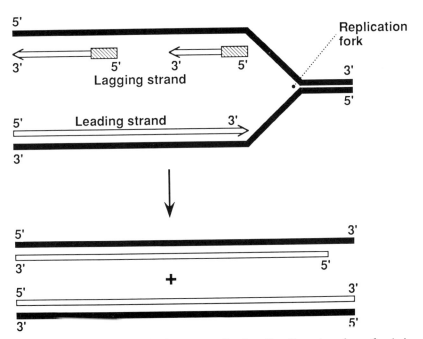

Fig. 7.16. The problem of telomere replication. Leading-strand synthesis is continuous to the telomere end. However, lagging-strand synthesis proceeds in segments using RNA primers (hatched) to initiate synthesis; these are subsequently removed and the DNA fragments are joined by the action of a polymerase. The lagging strand is thus shorter than its complementary 5' to 3' strand.

the 5′ to 3′ strand (the lagging strand) is carried out in segments of 1000 to 2000 base-pairs known as Okazaki fragments. Each Okazaki fragment starts with an RNA primer about 10 bp in length, which is subsequently removed as the fragments are linked to give the intact daughter strand.

The problem with this scenario occurs when the replication fork reaches the telomere. The leading strand can be synthesized right up to the telomere, but the lagging strand would be short by the length of the RNA primer needed to initiate the last Okazaki fragment. The unpaired section of the strand would be subject to nuclease degradation, and thus in each round of DNA replication the telomeres would be progressively whittled away.

It is now known that telomeres of all species have very similar structures, and consist of several hundred tandem repeats of a simple

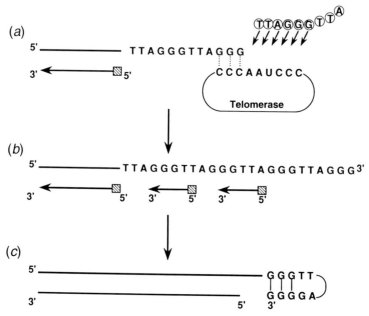

Fig. 7.17. Possible mode of action of telomerase. (*a*) The RNA sequence in telomerase pairs with nucleotides in the G-rich strand of DNA and provides a template for the stepwise addition of further bases of the repeat unit TTAGGG. (*b*) The C-rich strand is filled in by conventional lagging-strand synthesis. (*c*) The overhang in the G-rich strand forms non-Watson–Crick G–G bonds to stabilize the telomere ends.

sequence. The 5' to 3' strand towards the terminus is always rich in guanosine (G) residues, while the opposite strand is rich in cytosine (C) residues. In humans, the G-rich strand has a repeat unit (TTAGGG)$_n$ that overhangs the C-rich strand by 12 to 16 residues. There is evidence that this overhang may fold back on itself and be stabilized by non-Watson–Crick G-G base-pairing. (Watson–Crick base-pairing is always G·C and A·T). Such folded-back structures probably provide essential stability to chromosome ends.

There still remains the puzzle of telomere replication. The discovery of an enzyme, telomerase, has provided a coherent, though still incomplete, picture of the mechanics of this process. Telomerase is a terminal deoxynucleotidyl transferase capable of adding TTAGGG repeats, one nucleotide at a time, to the 3' end of the G-rich strand. The enzyme is a ribonucleoprotein complex containing an RNA sequence which both pairs with nucleotides in the G-rich strand and also acts as a template for addition of further bases (Fig. 7.17). The C-rich strand is then filled in by conventional lagging-strand synthesis. The maintenance of telomeres is thus a balanced process in which loss of DNA by conventional replication mechanisms is offset by sequential addition of nucleotides primed by the RNA template of telomerase.

This model for telomere replication suggests that telomerase is an essential enzyme in maintaining the full length of chromosomes. Analysis of telomere length as a function either of age or of the number of cell divisions shows a reduction in the mean number of TTAGGG repeats with the passage of time. Chromosomes in sperm and fetal tissues have an average of about 15 kb of repeats whereas in DNA from adult blood the average is about 10 kb. There is evidence that telomerase may be inactive in somatic tissues and that telomere length might be an indicator of the number of cell divisions that it has taken to form a particular tissue. It is not entirely fanciful to view ageing and senescence as a process in which the whittling away of the ends of chromosomes plays an important part.

DOWN SYNDROME

Down syndrome is the most common chromosomal abnormality in newborns, and also the most frequent genetic cause of mental retardation. The overall birth incidence is 1 in 800, but the older mother has a much higher risk, with a steep increase in incidence for mothers who are 35 or more years old. A majority of Down syndrome conceptions are spontaneously aborted, and thus risk figures depend on the stage of pregnancy at which ascertainment is made (Table 7.2).

Table 7.2. *Frequency of trisomy 21 in children and fetuses of older mothers*

Maternal age	Frequency of trisomy 21		
	At birth	At 16 weeks	At 12 weeks
35	1 in 380	1 in 300	1 in 240
37	1 in 240	1 in 190	1 in 130
39	1 in 150	1 in 120	1 in 75
41	1 in 85	1 in 70	1 in 40
43	1 in 50	1 in 40	1 in 25
45	1 in 28	1 in 22	1 in 13

For example, a 41-year-old mother has a risk of 1 in 85 of bearing a liveborn child with Down syndrome, but a higher risk of carrying a fetus if prenatal diagnosis is carried out at 16 weeks (1 in 70) or 12 weeks (1 in 40) of pregnancy. Exactly which risk should be quoted in counselling the older mother has been the subject of some controversy.

About 1% of Down syndrome patients are mosaics for trisomy 21 and a normal chromosome complement, and these tend to have a less severe phenotype.

arms of chromosomes 13, 14 or 15. The clinical phenotype is the same for trisomy 21 and translocation Down syndrome, with varying degrees of mental retardation and a spectrum of somatic abnormalities, of which the characteristic facies is the most prominent feature. About 1% of Down syndrome patients are mosaics for trisomy 21 and a normal chromosome complement, and these tend to have a less severe phenotype.

The origin of trisomy 21 is non-disjunction (failure of homologous chromosomes to separate at anaphase) during meiosis. Non-disjunction can occur either in oocytes (maternal non-disjunction) or in spermatocytes (paternal non-disjunction), and either at the first or at the second meiotic divisions (Fig. 7.18). When non-disjunction occurs at the second meiotic division, the trisomic individual inherits two copies of one of the parental chromosomes 21 and one copy of the other parental chromosome 21, whereas first division meiotic non-disjunction leads to three different parental chromosomes 21.

Study of chromosomal heteromorphisms, i.e. specific features of individual chromosomes visible under the light microscope, suggests that non-disjunction in the first meiotic division is the most common

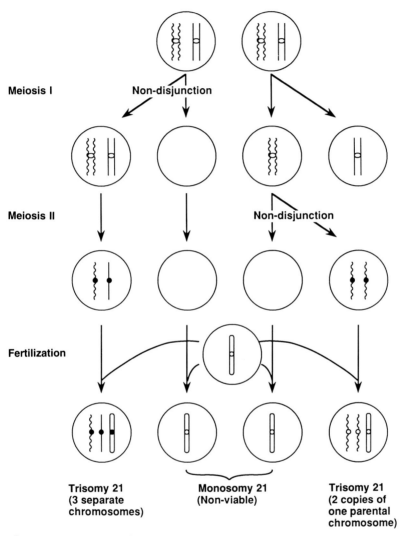

Fig. 7.18. The origin of trisomy 21 is non-disjunction of chromosomes 21 either at meiosis I or at meiosis II. The homologous chromosomes 21 in the cells at the top are represented by different configurations so that their origins in the zygotes (bottom row) can be traced. The cells at the top could be oocytes or spermatocytes but, in fact, are found to be oocytes in 95% of cases of trisomy 21.

cause of trisomy 21, and that in a large majority of cases this occurs in a maternal meiosis. Evaluation of heteromorphisms is, however, somewhat subjective. Investigation of polymorphic DNA markers is a more powerful technique, and has now shown that in 95% of cases of trisomy 21 the extra chromosome is of maternal origin. An example of this type of analysis is shown in Fig. 7.19. It must be noted that because of the possibility of recombination during meiosis, DNA markers cannot establish whether non-disjunction has occurred in the first or second meiotic division. No differences in clinical phenotype have been observed in Down syndrome cases with an extra paternal chromosome compared to those with an extra maternal chromosome.

The question of why an extra chromosome 21 causes the range of clinical features seen in Down syndrome continues to be a fascinating

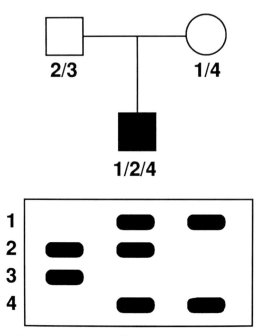

Fig. 7.19. The use of a multi-allelic DNA polymorphism to establish the origin of the extra chromosome 21 in a child with Down syndrome (filled square in pedigree). The father is heterozygous for bands 2 and 3 and the mother for bands 1 and 4. The affected child has inherited an extra chromosome 21 from his mother. See Fig. 7.11 for explanation of other symbols.

and unsolved issue. It is known from translocation cases and also from Down syndrome patients with only a partial trisomy that the critical region is part of the long arm of 21. Molecular genetic analysis has now begun to dissect this region. It would appear that many of the major phenotypic abnormalities of classic Down syndrome, such as the characteristic facies, hand anomalies (often clinodactyly of the fifth finger), congenital heart disease and some part of the mental retardation, reside in a duplication of q22.2 and part of q22.3 (Fig. 7.20). However, the rest of the long arm of chromosome 21 is clearly not irrelevant to the full-blown phenotype, and duplication of genes in the q11 to q22.1 region undoubtedly contribute to the extent of mental retardation, and perhaps to other more variable features found in some but not all cases of Down syndrome.

There is little doubt that discovery of further partial trisomies and translocations of chromosome 21 will produce a more refined map of the correlation between duplicated genes and clinical phenotype. As yet, however, there is little understanding of why extra copies of genes so unbalance cellular mechanisms. There is considerable evidence that specific enzymes whose genetic loci have been mapped

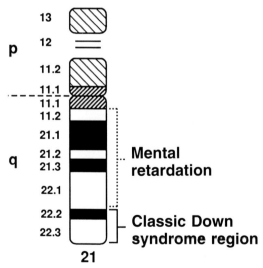

Fig. 7.20. A schematic representation of chromosome 21 showing the duplicated region leading to the classic Down syndrome phenotype and an additional region, which may be responsible for more variable features.

to chromosome 21q are present at about 50% higher level in cells and tissues from Down syndrome patients. Data from non-enzymatic proteins is still lacking. None the less, the concept of gene dosage effects having an impact on cells during critical phases of differentiation and development is likely to remain central to the unravelling of the puzzle of the Down syndrome phenotype.

THE FRAGILE X SYNDROME

X-linked patterns of inheritance of mental retardation have been known for many years. In fact, the 1990 edition of McKusick's *Mendelian Inheritance in Man* lists 179 validated conditions with X-linked inheritance, about a quarter of which have variable associations with mental handicap. However, it was not until 1969 that a clearcut syndrome was established in which X-linked mental retardation segregated with a marker chromosome. The cytogenetic benchmark of this condition, now known as the Martin–Bell or fragile X syndrome, is a non-staining gap on the long arm of the X chromosome at Xq27.3 (Fig. 7.21). The site is not detected under ordinary culture conditions, but needs special media with folate depletion or thymidine excess before it shows up. Even then the fragile site is rarely visible in more than 50% of mitotic cells from affected individuals.

The key clinical features of the fragile X syndrome in males are moderate to severe mental retardation, a long face with large everted

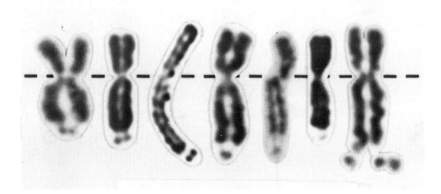

Fig. 7.21. Variation in appearance of human X chromosomes expressing the fragile site at Xq27.3 in peripheral blood cells cultured in folate-depleted medium, or in medium containing excess thymidine to inhibit thymidylate synthetase. Courtesy of Dr Christine Gosden.

ears (Fig. 7.22) and large testes. Although defined cytogenetically, it is in essence a Mendelian condition, albeit one with some very peculiar features. Some 30% to 50% of obligate female carriers also show a degree of mental retardation or impairment. Carriers who are mentally retarded usually score positive for the fragile site on cytogenetic examination, whereas most carriers who are mentally normal lack the fragile site. These observations are consistent with X-linked dominant inheritance with incomplete penetrance. However, more detailed examination of the segregation pattern of the fragile X syndrome reveals complexities and inconsistencies that cannot be easily reconciled with inheritance of a single mutation.

The most startling of these is the pattern of transmission of the syndrome by normal males. Such men, who may be demonstrated by pedigree analysis (Fig. 7.23) to be transmitters, never have affected daughters. However, their grandchildren (both males and females) are often affected. This gives rise to the concept of a premutation being converted to a full mutation only after passage through female meiosis. Since the full fragile X syndrome is the most common source of inherited mental retardation (1 in 1500 males, 1 in 2000 females), carriers of the premutation are likely to be remarkably frequent.

Over the past few years there have been intense efforts to clone the fragile X site. This was initially frustrated by the immense size of what

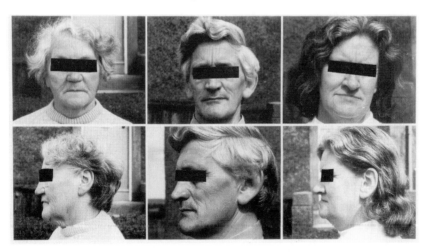

Fig. 7.22. An unaffected but fragile-X-positive mother (left) and her affected son (centre) and daughter (right). Note the long forehead, large jaw and large ears in the affected son and daughter. Courtesy of Dr Christine Gosden.

is a cytogenetically visible region and even the closest markers showed a high rate of recombination with the syndrome. The advent of megabase cloning techniques in the form of pulsed-field gel electrophoresis and yeast artificial chromosomes (YACs) speeded the search, and soon several groups reported individual YAC clones containing bracketing markers and therefore (in the absence of chromosome rearrangements) presumed to encompass the fragile site. This culminated in May 1991 with a series of reports describing a gene (FMR-1) now believed to be responsible for the fragile X syndrome.

The properties of FMR-1 go some way towards unravelling the extraordinary genetics of fragile X mental retardation and its other phenotypic effects. The most unusual feature is an unstable region of DNA represented by a CGG repeat in a 5′ exon of the gene. This trinucleotide, which codes for arginine, shows a remarkable degree of length variation. Normal males and females have between 6 and 54 copies of the repeat with a median value at about 30. Phenotypically normal transmitting males and normal carrier females have a premu-

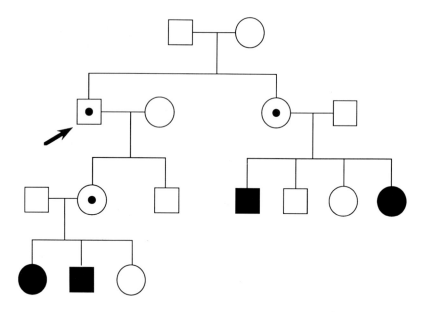

Fig. 7.23. Typical pedigree seen in the fragile X syndrome. Affected individuals are represented by filled symbols; symbols representing premutation carriers have a central dot. A normal transmitting male is arrowed.

tation, where the copy number of the CGG repeat has been expanded to between 60 and 200. The premutation is stable in male meiosis and is transmitted without change in copy number. But it is unstable in female meiosis, and often leads to an enormous increase in copy number, and the development of the full-blown fragile X syndrome in both the sons and daughters of transmitting females. The risk of a female premutation carrier having an affected son depends on the size of her repeat unit; at more than 140 repeats there is almost invariable expansion to a full mutation, and a boy inheriting this X chromosome will have fragile X syndrome.

The presence of a premutation in a male or female may be detected by Southern blotting and demonstration of a fragment of increased size on a gel (Fig. 7.24). The full mutation is detected as a smear in the high molecular weight region. Methods have now been developed for PCR amplification of the CGG region, which permits more accurate estimates of copy number, and may well soon be applied to wide-scale screening of carriers of this important source of mental retardation.

CONTIGUOUS GENE SYNDROMES

At the highest resolution, light microscopy is capable of resolving a chromosomal deletion or duplication of about 2000 kb of genomic DNA, but this cannot be achieved systematically and much depends on the quality of the chromosome spread. In many chromosomal syndromes, cytogenetically visible aberrations are not observed consistently and the reasonable assumption has been made that the microscopically invisible cases represent smaller alterations in part of the same material. A case in point is the Prader–Willi syndrome, referred to earlier, where only about 50% of patients have a visible interstitial deletion of 15q11–q13.

Use of molecular genetic technology has begun to bridge the gap between conventional chromosome disorders and single gene defects. Pulsed-field gel electrophoresis and routine restriction mapping has permitted the description of a new type of abnormality, the contiguous gene syndrome, in which several adjacent genes are altered simultaneously. It is not a particularly precise term, since it has been used to cover conditions in which some patients have visible cytogenetic abnormalities whereas others do not, as well as conditions in which no visible chromosome aberration has yet been detected. In some contiguous gene syndromes the nature of the deleted genes is fairly exactly known, while in others the genes involved in the affected region are largely unknown. It must therefore be remembered that contiguous gene syndrome is a provisional classification likely to undergo revision and evolution.

Roy Schmickel, who coined the term contiguous gene syndrome in 1986, restricted it to retinoblastoma, Wilms' tumour/Beckwith–Wiedemann syndrome, and the Prader–Willi, Langer–Giedion, Miller–Diecker and DiGeorge syndromes. The first two of these were discussed in Chapter 6, and the Prader–Willi (and related Angelman) syndromes earlier in this chapter. Several other contiguous gene syndromes are listed in Table 7.3. All can occur as de novo events or, less

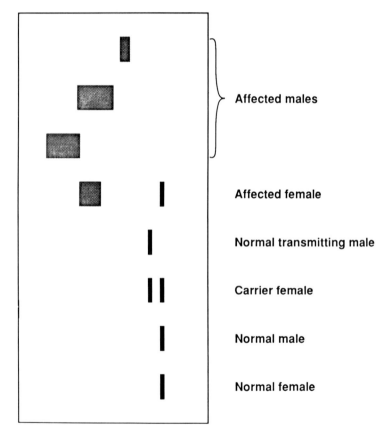

Fig. 7.24. Southern blot patterns seen on probing for the association between the numbers of CGG repeats and the fragile X syndrome. In both affected males and affected females the full mutation is detected as a somewhat variable smear of high molecular weight DNA fragments.

Table 7.3. *Contiguous gene syndromes*

Syndrome	Chromosomal region affected
Langer–Giedion	8q24 deletions
WAGR	11p13 deletions
Beckwith–Wiedemann	11p15 duplications
Retinoblastoma	13q14 deletions
Prader–Willi, Angelman	15q11 deletions
Miller–Diecker	17p13 deletions
DiGeorge	22q11 deletions

frequently, as Mendelian conditions. In each case, analysis of patients carrying microscopically visible cytogenetic aberrations has pinpointed the chromosomal region that is worth further exploration by molecular techniques.

An example of molecular mapping in a contiguous gene syndrome is provided by the Miller–Diecker syndrome (MDS). In this rare disorder, patients have a characteristic facies – short nose with upturned nares, bitemporal grooving of a high forehead, prominent upper lip and micrognathia – as well as retarded postnatal growth and severe mental retardation. Death occurs in early childhood and the most striking post-mortem feature is lissencephaly, a smooth brain without convolutions or gyri. MDS was first thought to be an autosomal recessive condition, because of occasional recurrence in siblings of an affected case. Subsequently a number of patients were found in whom a subtle microdeletion had occurred of the tip of the short arm of chromosome 17, a G-band-negative region, which makes precise mapping difficult. This stimulated a search, using DNA probes, for evidence of microdeletions in 'non-chromosomal' cases of MDS. It is now possible to build up a consensus picture of the critical MDS region, showing the smallest region of overlap to be an interstitial deletion of about 100 kb (Fig. 7.25).

Studies of this type in MDS and other contiguous gene syndromes go some way towards explaining the phenotypic variation in different patients. Large deletions, even when microscopically invisible, are more likely to lead to a severe phenotype. They also make it possible to begin to pinpoint functional genes in the deletion regions and their possible roles in contributing to specific symptoms. For example, the gene for profilin, an actin-binding protein, is deleted in some but not

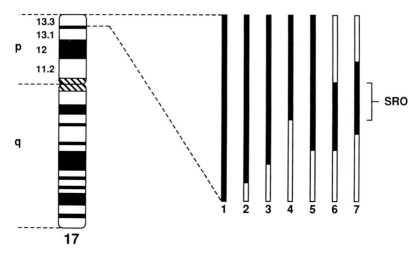

Fig. 7.25. A consensus map of the MDS region at 17p13. Analysis of DNA polymorphisms in patients with differing extents of deletion of 17p (indicated by seven cases at the right: filled boxes represent the deletions) have permitted definition of the smallest region of overlap (SRO) of about 100 kb.

all cases of MDS, and thus must be seen as possibly contributing to, but certainly not essential to, the phenotype. Furthermore, the expanding sensitivity of DNA probing for deletions and rearrangements also opens up the possibility of examining the parents of contiguous gene syndrome cases for submicroscopic, balanced chromosome translocations. Apparent de novo cases are not necessarily new mutations, and might instead be the result of malsegregation of unrecognized balanced translocations.

SUGGESTED READING

Antonarakis, S. E., Lewis, J. G., Adelsberger, P. A., Peterson, M. B., Schinzel, A. A., Binkert, F., *et al.* (1991). Parental origin of the extra chromosome in trisomy 21 as indicated by analysis of DNA polymorphisms. *New England Journal of Medicine* **324**: 872–876.

Berta, P., Hawkins, J. R., Sinclair, A. H., Taylor, A., Griffiths, B. L., Goodfellow, P. N. and Fellous, M. (1990). Genetic evidence equating SRY and the testis-determining factor. *Nature (London)* **348**: 448–450.

Blackburn, E. H. (1991). Structure and function of telomeres. *Nature (London)* **350**: 569–573.

Brown, C. J., Ballabio, A., Rupert, J. L., Lafreniere, R. G., Grompe, M., Tonlorenzi, R. and Willard, H. F. (1991*a*). A gene from the region of the human X inactivation centre is expressed exclusively from the inactive X chromosome. *Nature (London)* **349**: 38–44.

Brown, C. J., Lafreniere, R. G., Powers, V. E., Sebastio, G., Ballabio, A., Pettigrew, A. L., *et al.* (1991*b*). Localisation of the X-inactivation centre on the human X chromosome in Xq13. *Nature (London)* **349**: 82–84.

Davies, K. E. (Editor), (1989). *The Fragile X Syndrome*. Oxford University Press, Oxford.

De la Chapelle, A. (1988). Invited editorial: the complicated issue of human sex determination. *American Journal of Human Genetics* **43**: 1–3.

Emanuel, B. S. (1988). Invited editorial: molecular cytogenetics: towards dissection of the contiguous gene syndromes. *American Journal of Human Genetics* **43**: 575–578.

Epstein C. J. (1990). The consequences of chromosome imbalance. *American Journal of Medical Genetics, supplement* **7**: 31–37.

Ferguson-Smith, M. A. (1991). Invited editorial: putting the genetics back into cytogenetics. *American Journal of Human Genetics* **48**: 179–182.

Greider, C. W. (1990). Telomere, telomerase and senescense. *Bioessays* **12**: 363–369.

Hall, J. G. (1990). Genomic imprinting: review and relevance to human diseases. *American Journal of Human Genetics* **46**: 857–873.

Hastie, N. D. and Allshire, R. C. (1989). Human telomeres: fusion and interstitial sites. *Trends in Genetics* **5**: 326–330.

Jäger, R. J., Anvret, M., Hall, K. and Scherer, G. (1990). A human XY female with a frameshift mutation in the candidate testes-determining gene, SRY. *Nature (London)* **348**: 452–454.

Koopman, P., Gubbay, J., Vivien, N., Goodfellow, P. and Lovell-Badge, R. (1991). Male development of chromosomally female mice transgenic for SRY. *Nature (London)* **351**: 117–121.

Korenberg, J. R., Kawashima, H., M.-Pulst, S., Allen, L., Magenis, E. and Epstein, C. J. (1990). Down syndrome: towards a molecular definition of the phenotype. *American Journal of Medical Genetics, supplement* **7**: 91–97.

Lyon, M. F. (1988). X chromosome inactivation and the location and expression of X-linked genes. *American Journal of Human Genetics* **42**: 8–16.

Lyon, M. F. (1991). The quest for the X inactivation centre. *Trends in Genetics* **7**: 69–70.

207

Oberlé, I., Rousseau, F., Heitz, D., Kretz, C., Devys, D., Hanauer, A., *et al.* (1991). Instability of a 550-base pair DNA segment and abnormal methylation in fragile X syndrome. *Science* **252**: 1097–1102.

Reik, W. (1989). Genomic imprinting and genetic disorders in man. *Trends in Genetics* **5**: 331–336.

Sapienza, C. (1991). Genome imprinting and carcinogenesis. *Biochmica et Biophysica Acta* **1072**: 51–61.

Schmickel, R. D. (1986). Contiguous gene syndromes: a component of recognizable syndromes. *Journal of Pediatrics* **109**: 231–241.

Trask, B. J. (1991). Fluorescence in situ hybridization. *Trends in Genetics* **7**: 149–154.

Verkerk, A. J. M. H., Pieretti, M., Sutcliffe, J. S., Fu, Y.-H., Kuhl, D. P. A., Pizzuti, A., *et al.* (1991). Identification of a gene (FMR-1) containing a CGG repeat coincident with a break-point cluster region exhibiting length variation in fragile X syndrome. *Cell* **65**: 905–914.

Yu, S., Pritchard, M., Kremer, E., Lynch, M., Nancarrow, J., Baker, E., *et al.* (1991). Fragile X genotype characterized by an unstable region of DNA. *Science* **252**: 1179–1181.

8 MULTIFACTORIAL DISORDERS

As pointed out in Chapter 2, most of the common human diseases, as well as a majority of serious congenital malformations seen in the newborn, are not caused by mutant genes at a single genetic locus. Some of these diseases may be polygenic, resulting from the interaction of several genes, each with a comparatively minor effect, but whose consequences are additive. It is more likely that many also involve an interplay of genes and environmental factors, so that the aggregate of causative effects is best referred to as multifactorial. Traditional genetic analysis has not been particularly successful in tackling multifactorial disorders, because of the complexity of the probable interactions between genes and the environment. Even the analysis of concordance rates for a disorder between monozygotic and dizygotic twins (see Table 2.6) does little more than rank disorders in terms of the probable importance of a genetic versus an environmental aetiology.

The spectacular success of molecular genetics in tackling Mendelian disorders obviously raises the hope that the same technologies might be applied to the more complicated, and more common, multifactorial disorders. The objectives of such approaches are, however, likely to be slightly different. Understanding the nature of the mutant gene responsible for cystic fibrosis, for example, will, in the fullness of time, be expected to explain a very large part of the clinical and pathological consequences of that disorder, as well as providing an immediate handle for prenatal diagnosis and carrier detection. The discovery of a mutant gene that appears to be part of the pathology of a disorder such as diabetes will, however, be only a beginning of an understanding of the whole disorder process, and may have little immediate effect on either diagnosis or prevention. But such is the power of molecular genetics that it will be an enormously important beginning. The ability to deduce the structure and function of the protein product of most genes that have been sequenced is a very powerful weapon for starting to disentangle the biochemistry of even the most complicated disorders. It can be seen as the first ray of light in a sea of darkness, which we hope will be followed by further rays of light until the whole subject is comprehensively illuminated.

The key words in the above sentence are 'we hope' and 'illuminated'. There is as yet little direct evidence that the molecular genetic approach to multifactorial disorders will succeed where more traditional approaches have failed. The hope rests on the undoubted fact that molecular technologies are the most powerful yet to be applied to biological problems, and that the scope and range of the techniques used is still evolving. Although some doubts remain about just how successful these approaches will be, they must be viewed within the gathering momentum of mapping and then sequencing the entire human genome (Chapter 9). As the number of DNA marker systems increases remorselessly, it will become progressively easier to tie even the most complex disorder into cloned sequences of known or inferred function.

The primary purpose of this endeavour will be, in the first instance, to illuminate the biology of specific disorders. This point needs to be made because much of the early clinical success of molecular genetics has been directed towards prenatal diagnosis of Mendelian disorders. This has tended to leave the unfortunate impression that DNA analysis is concerned with search-and-destroy functions. It is both inevitable and right that the technical ability to detect fetuses with severe disorders should be pressed into clinical service as soon as possible. But it has tended to overshadow the even greater ability of molecular genetics as a technology for dissecting the workings of both normal and mutant genes. Amongst the multifactorial disorders, where understanding is likely to lead to management, treatment and even cure, this misconception will eventually be corrected.

There should be no illusions about the difficulties confronting the molecular geneticist investigating multifactorial disorders. The lack of diagnostic specificity, genuine heterogeneity within named disorders, variable ages of onset (so that unaffecteds may be not yet affected) and the unknown modifying effect of the environment are just a few of the problems. The frontal assault, so successful in Mendelian disorders, is inappropriate. But, as this chapter attempts to indicate, simplifying assumptions and piecemeal approaches are beginning to yield some useful results.

DISEASE ASSOCIATIONS

The study of associations between particular diseases and genetic polymorphisms has a long history, reaching back to the 1920s and the years following the discovery of the ABO blood group system. The

Table 8.1. *Some significant HLA and disease associations*

Disease	Increased HLA antigen(s)
Acute anterior uveitis	B27
Ankylosing spondylitis	B27
Behcet disease	B5
Coeliac disease	B8, DR3, DR7
Dermatitis herpetiformis	B8, DR3
Goodpasture syndrome	DR2
Grave's disease	B8, DR3
Haemochromatosis	A3, B7, B14
Insulin-dependent diabetes mellitus	B8, B15, DR3, DR4
Multiple sclerosis	B7, DR2
Myasthenia gravis	B8
Narcolepsy	DR2
Psoriasis	B13, B17, B37, CW6, DR7
Pemphigus vulgaris	A26, B38, DR4
Reiter disease	B27
Rheumatoid arthritis	B27, DR4
Sjögren syndrome	B8, DW3
Systemic lupus erythematosus	B8, DR3

Source: From Tiwari, J. and Terasaki, P. (1985) *HLA and Disease Associations.* Springer–Verlag, New York.

association between blood group O and duodenal ulcer as well as that between blood group A and cancer of the stomach are now well-established examples of this phenomenon, but at one time almost every common disease was claimed by some investigator to show a statistically significant association with a particular blood group. However, the inability to find any biological explanation for such associations gradually discouraged further collections of data, and it was not until the discovery of the highly polymorphic major histocompatibility complex (or HLA complex) that association studies re-emerged as an approach to the analysis of susceptibility genes in man. Not only are the associations between HLA specificities and certain diseases much stronger than those seen with blood group antigens, but there is an obvious connection between the role of the major histocompatibility complex in mediating the immune response and an autoimmune aetiology in many of the associated diseases (Table 8.1).

The advent of molecular genetic techniques has greatly increased the potential of disease-association studies. In the first place it has introduced a whole new set of genetic markers, many of which are highly polymorphic. It has also extended the range of alleles making up existing polymorphic loci. This aspect is a particular feature of the HLA complex, whose extensive array of serologically defined antigens has been subdivided and redefined by molecular typing using the polymerase chain reaction. A map of the alleles at the class I and class II regions of the HLA complex is shown in Fig. 8.1. Although at first sight this seems an impossibly complicated system, it is simplified by the fact that the entire HLA complex covers only about 3 Mb (3000 kb) of genomic DNA, so that cross-overs between alleles at the constituent loci are comparatively rare. Extended haplotypes, constructed by typing for alleles at the different loci, tend to be inherited as highly informative discrete units. The HLA complex is on the short arm of chromosome 6 and thus individuals inherit one extended haplotype from each of their parents (Fig. 8.2).

The study of disease associations is conventionally carried out by comparing the frequency of a polymorphic allele in a patient group to the frequency in a control group drawn from the same population. The null hypothesis is that the frequencies in the two groups will not differ significantly. When they do differ, the relative risk (or relative incidence) can be calculated as shown in Table 8.2; this indicates how many times more frequent the disease is in individuals with a specific

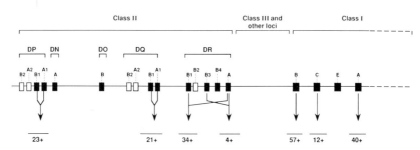

Fig. 8.1. Map of loci in the HLA region. Expressing genes are represented by filled boxes and non-expressing or pseudogenes by open boxes. In the class II region, genes are expressed as αβ-heterodimers with the α-chain coded for by the A gene and the β-chain coded for by the B gene. Most of the polymorphism resides in the β-chains. Approximate minimum number of alleles for each system is shown at bottom.

212

Table 8.2. *Calculation of relative risk*

	Numbers of individuals	
	B27-positive	B27-negative
Patients with ankylosing spondylitis	180	20
Controls	35	465

$$\text{Relative risk} = \frac{180}{35} \div \frac{20}{465} = 120$$

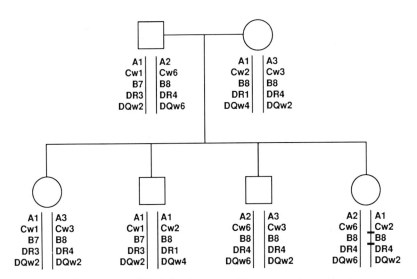

Fig. 8.2. Inheritance of HLA haplotypes. The parental origin of each chromosome in the first three children can be identified. In the fourth child a recombinant chromosome (marked by cross-bars) has been inherited from the child's mother.

213

marker allele than in individuals without it. Statistically significant deviations from the null hypothesis are evidence for an association between a particular allele and a particular disease. However, there are many traps for the unwary. Patient and control groups must be carefully matched both socially and geographically, since many marker systems show dramatic differences in allele frequencies in quite closely related subpopulations. Mutation rates at both the marker locus and the hypothetical disease-susceptibility locus must be low, or genuine associations will be obscured. The significance of any discovered association must be modulated by the number of marker systems examined; a p-value of 0.05 is significant if a single system has been examined, but for ten marker systems a p-value of 0.005 is required before the claim of statistical significance can be made.

The difficulty with disease-association studies is knowing how to interpret them. Very few associations have been discovered of sufficient magnitude to be of practical value in risk estimation. One exception that pre-dates molecular technology is the association between ankylosing spondylitis and the HLA–B27 allele (Table 8.1). Individuals with this allele are about 100 times more likely to develop ankylosing spondylitis than those with other HLA–B alleles, and this suggests that the HLA–B locus is a major genetic determinant of the disease. However, in most other disease associations, relative risks are comparatively modest. This might occur because the marker locus has a genuine but relatively minor contribution to susceptibility, while other genes and environmental factors are more important determinants of disease. Alternatively the association might be the result of linkage disequilibrium, with the apparently predisposing locus genetically linked to an as yet undiscovered susceptibility locus. An example of this is to be found in reports of associations between insulin-dependent diabetes mellitus and antigens encoded by the class I HLA–A and HLA–B loci. It is now apparent that these associations are the result of linkage disequilibrium within the extended HLA region, and that major determinants of genetic susceptibility map more closely to the class II HLA–D region (see Fig. 8.1).

It obviously makes sense when studying disease associations to concentrate on marker loci that encode proteins that might have some phenotypic relationship to the disease. Thus the study of HLA association with autoimmune-type disease makes some biological sense, as do associations between genes involved in lipid metabolism and cardiovascular disease. But even when statistically significant associations are found, this must be seen as little more than a starting point.

In the final analysis the definition of a susceptibility gene depends on some form of linkage analysis.

LINKAGE ANALYSIS

In moving to linkage analysis of complex disorders, one is confronted by the problem that there is seldom any clear pattern of inheritance enabling the cosegregation of marker and disease loci to be analysed by the methods outlined in Chapter 5. Even when allowance is made for diagnostic uncertainties (e.g. at what point does high blood pressure become essential hypertension?), disease heterogeneity (e.g. is schizophrenia one or several disorders?) and variable age of onset (e.g. is Alzheimer's disease part of a normal ageing process?), many of these disorders are probably polygenic, so that a defined mode of inheritance cannot be assigned in tracking marker systems. Mathematical models attempting to handle the segregation of several causative gene loci are very complex, and even so must make untestable assumptions about epistatic effects (the effect of one gene or gene product on another gene or gene product). The progress that has been made in mathematical treatment of multi-locus disorders, though showing promise in organisms that may be used in breeding experiments, has yet to be applied with any success in human genetics. None the less, there seems little doubt that once a reasonable map of the human genome is produced these complex treatments will begin to yield results.

For the present, linkage analysis in multifactorial disorders has to employ simplifying procedures. These include sibling-pair analysis, random mapping of major genes in subsets of the disorder showing Mendelian modes of segregation, candidate-gene linkage analysis and mutation analysis in genes thought to have a major impact on the disease. Although each of these topics is discussed separately below, several of these approaches are often applied simultaneously in the more important multifactorial disorders.

SIBLING-PAIR ANALYSIS

As long ago as 1935 Lionel Penrose noted that evidence of linkage could be obtained from data on a single generation of a family if concordance of disease status and a marker system were analysed on multiple sets of pairs of siblings. Consider the example in Table 8.3. Siblings are either like or unlike for the particular disease, and like or unlike for the specific marker being tested – a protein or DNA polymorphism. In the absence of linkage between marker and disease there should be equal proportions of siblings in each column of Table

Table 8.3. *Sibling-pair analysis for a disease and marker system*

		Disease status	
		Siblings like	Siblings unlike
Marker system	Siblings like	a	c
	Siblings unlike	b	d
In the absence of linkage		$\dfrac{a}{a+b} = \dfrac{c}{c+d}$	
In the presence of linkage		$\dfrac{a}{a+b}$ significantly different from $\dfrac{c}{c+d}$	

8.3. If, however, the marker is linked to a major locus responsible for at least some part of the disease phenotype, there may be significant deviations from the expected ratios. No assumption is made about the mode of inheritance of the disease.

There are many disadvantages in this type of analysis. Absence of information on the marker status of the parents means that informative and uninformative matings cannot be separated, so that informative matings may represent a small fraction of the total. Even if there is tight linkage between marker and disease, the deviation from independence may be small and can be simulated by confounding effects such as disease heterogeneity. Furthermore, in adult-onset disorders unaffected siblings may actually be not yet affected siblings. None the less, the first autosomal linkage defined in humans, that between Lutheran and Lewis blood groups, was detected in this way.

One way of avoiding the problem of possible late onset is to conduct the analysis on only affected sibling pairs and to classify the pairs on the basis of haplotype sharing. For an autosomal marker system, affected pairs will have: (a) both haplotypes identical; or (b) one haplotype identical; or (c) neither haplotype identical. The prior expectation for a marker unlinked to the disease locus is a frequency distribution of 0.25, 0.5 and 0.25, respectively, for the three categories above. Table 8.4 shows an analysis of sibling-pairs affected with insulin-dependent diabetes mellitus for haplotype sharing at the HLA and insulin gene loci. No deviation was seen from expected ratios at the insulin gene locus. However, significant deviation at the HLA locus suggests a major diabetic gene linked to the HLA complex, a conclusion supported by a variety of other studies.

216

Table 8.4. *Haplotype sharing at the HLA and insulin gene (IG) loci in affected sibling-pairs with insulin-dependent diabetes mellitus*

	% of pairs sharing haplotypes		
	2	1	0
HLA locus	59	34	7
IG locus	24	52	24
Expectation (no linkage)	25	50	25

Source: From Cox and Spielman (1989).

Affected sibling-pair analysis is a fairly robust screening tool for linkage because it requires no model of the mode of inheritance. It can be modified to take account of variable age of onset and of more than two affected members in a large sibling relationship. One important extension is based on the fact that it is more striking for affected distant relatives in a family (e.g. cousins) to share a rare marker allele than it is for them to share a common marker allele, and this is referred to as the affected-pedigree-member analysis. All these modifications require quite sophisticated mathematical treatments. What is important is that they are screening tools for preliminary evidence of linkage to susceptibility loci, rather than demonstrations that linkage may be taken for granted. In most instances, the investigator will wish to follow such preliminary findings by a full analysis of putative cosegregation of a marker and a disease in an extended multi-generational family.

RANDOM LINKAGE ANALYSIS OF MENDELIAN FORMS OF A COMPLEX DISORDER

One avenue to linkage analysis that is currently finding considerable favour in the analysis of complex disorders is the seeking out of groups of families in which segregation of the disease appears to follow a Mendelian pattern. I have already discussed applications of this approach in the chapter on cancer genetics. Dominantly inherited cancer syndromes (see Table 6.1) have been of inestimable value in focusing on and eventually isolating cancer-susceptibility genes, which are thought to have a major role in the more common multifactorial forms of the same (or even different) cancers. This is sometimes termed the reductionist approach, the philosophy being to reduce a

Table 8.5. *Classification of mental retardation*

Classification	I.Q. range	Alternative classification	Population percentage
Mild	50–70	Mild	2–3%
Moderate	35–50 ⎫		
Severe	20–35 ⎬	Severe	0.4%
Profound	0–20 ⎭		

complex problem to those elements for which there is a practical solution and then to hope that the specific solutions will be relevant to the more general problem.

In many common disorders it is possible to find and collect families in which segregation appears to be as an autosomal dominant, autosomal recessive or X-linked recessive. If a single large family or smaller sets of families are available, all showing the same mode of inheritance, linkage analysis can be carried out using panels of probes detecting DNA sequence polymorphisms. Such random mapping is tedious and time consuming, but is occasionally spectacularly successful. It obviously helps if an X-linked subset of families can be found, for this limits the exercise to a single small chromosome abundantly endowed with DNA polymorphisms.

Mental retardation
Mental retardation is classified within approximate I.Q. ranges (Table 8.5), a broad division placing severe mental retardation in the range of 0 to 50 and mild mental retardation in the range 50–70. The former has an estimated incidence of about 0.4%, while the latter comprises between 2% and 3% of the population. In both groups males consistently outnumber females, the excess being greatest for mild mental retardation. It has long been suspected that major genetic loci related to intellectual functioning are located on the X chromosome and operate as X-linked recessives. Estimates for the population prevalence of X-linked mental retardation have suggested that up to 20 separate loci may be involved. This is probably a considerable underestimate.

Inspection of McKusick's *Mendelian Inheritance in Man* (1990) shows in the X-linked catalogue some 70 diagnostic entities in which mental retardation is an associated feature. Many of these are distinct syndromes with reasonably clear defining clinical manifestations, such as macrocephaly, microcephaly, dysmorphic features, skeletal anomalies, visual dysfunction or deafness. There still remains an excess of male mental retardation, referred to as non-syndromal or non-specific, that represents a considerable problem to the genetic counsellor. Once the relatively common fragile X syndrome has been excluded, the recurrence risk to the brother of an isolated male proband with severe idiopathic mental retardation is about one in six, and for a male proband with mild idiopathic mental retardation about one in four. Both figures suggest either heterogeneity within defined but unknown X-linked Mendelian conditions, or multifactorial inheritance.

In view of the fact that the X chromosome represents only about 6% of the human genome, it has made sense to concentrate, in the first instance, on random mapping of mental retardation to this chromosome. Fig. 8.3 shows the progress that has been made in regional assignments of Mendelian conditions associated with X-linked mental retardation and indicates the considerable size of the problem. Even simple non-syndromal X-linked mental retardation (XLMR) maps to three or four distinct regions of the chromosome, and almost inevitably will turn out not to be the consequence of mutations at single loci. Only in the fragile X syndrome has there been success in identifying and cloning the relevant gene (Chapter 7), and this is due almost entirely to the associated cytogenetic abnormality. However, both genetic and physical mapping of the X chromosome is proceeding at an accelerating pace, and it is reasonable to expect the cloning of other genes associated with both severe and mild mental retardation in the near future.

Epilepsy
In the absence of X-linkage, random mapping is a more formidable process, but by no means impossible. Again, it is a great help if a complex disorder can be dissected into Mendelian subgroups and then these attacked systematically. Recently there has been progress in applying this strategy to epilepsy. The epileptic disorders are clinically and aetiologically heterogeneous, a recent classification listing a total of 18 different varieties of seizure and 48 distinguishable clinical types. Amongst these, Mendelian disorders account for probably fewer than 1% of cases, and even here there are perhaps only two pure monogenic epilepsy syndromes – benign familial neonatal convulsions and progressive myoclonic epilepsy of the Unverricht–Lundborg type.

Benign familial neonatal convulsions is inherited as an autosomal

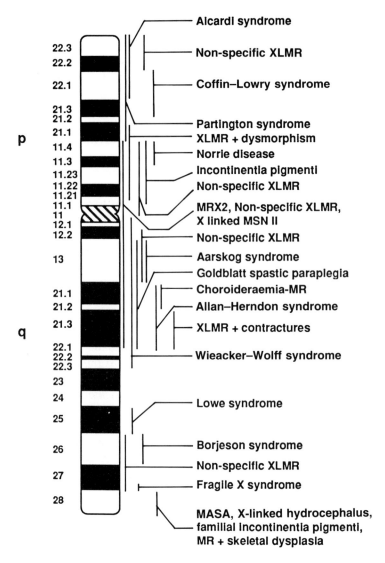

Fig. 8.3. Regional assignments, to the X chromosome, of Mendelian disorders associated with mental retardation. Note that there are at least four regions of non-syndromal X-linked mental retardation. From Glass (1991).

dominant with high penetrance. Random mapping of a set of families with 96 DNA markers has given strong evidence of linkage to the long arm of chromosome 20. Progressive myoclonic epilepsy of the Unverricht–Lundborg type is an autosomal recessive with a relatively high incidence in the Finnish population. Systematic testing of some 64 markers on families with several affected siblings excluded some 25% of the genome before linkage was established to the long arm of chromosome 21. In each of these two disorders there were no prior clues to the chromosomal localization of the relevant genes, and they must be seen as examples of successful application of the 'sweat and tears' approach to linkage analysis.

Psychotic illness

One should not underestimate the difficulties of random mapping of complex disorders, particularly when diagnostic criteria are ill defined. Nowhere is this better illustrated than in attempts to obtain genetic linkage to the two major groups of psychoses, bipolar affective illness (manic depression) and schizophrenia. Each of these groups of disorders has a population prevalence in developed countries that approaches 1%, and in each there is impressive evidence for familial aggregations. In manic depression, the risk to first-degree relatives is between 5% and 10%, while the concordance rate for monozygotic twins is almost 80%. In schizophrenia, the risk to first-degree relatives is of the order of 10%, while the monozygotic-twin concordance rate is about 50%. Both conditions are a major public health problem and represent baffling phenomena at the molecular and cellular level.

Apparent X-linkage of some families with manic depression has been reported on numerous occasions, particularly amongst groups of non-Ashkenazi Jewish origin. Segregation patterns are consistent with X-linked dominant inheritance. Linkage to glucose-6-phosphate dehydrogenase and both protan and deutan colour blindness placed the susceptibility locus in the Xq28 region. However, a separate study on a set of Belgian families gave evidence of linkage to the coagulation factor IX gene, which maps to Xq27, some 30 to 40 centimorgans from the glucose-6-phosphate dehydrogenase/colour blindness complex. Thus at least two putative X-linked genes may be involved. To complicate matters further, a study of manic depression in the tightly knit, old order Amish community of Pennsylvania showed cosegregation with the insulin and H-*ras*-1 genes, both of which map to the short arm of chromosome 11. Chromosome 11 linkage has not been confirmed in other populations, or indeed in the old order Amish

221

Table 8.6. *Tentative hints of genetic linkage in the major psychoses*

Psychoses	Chromosomal region of possible linkage
Manic depressive illness	11p
	Xq27
	Xq28
Schizophrenia	5q11–q13

population when re-examined. A change in clinical studies of two members of the original pedigree and inclusion of an additional branch of the family changed a lod score of greater than 4 to a negative value.

The situation in schizophrenia is even more doubtful, perhaps because diagnostic criteria are less certain than they are in manic depression. Linkage studies in this disorder began with an important clue: the cosegregation of a partial trisomy of a 20 to 30 centimorgan region of chromosome 5 (5q11.2–q13.3) with two affected individuals in an Asian family. This region was believed (incorrectly) to harbour the glucocorticoid receptor (GRL) gene, and since steroid psychosis resembles schizophrenia in some ways, GRL was an excellent candidate gene. This was followed by a demonstration of linkage between two markers in the 5q region defined by the trisomy in several British and Icelandic schizophrenia families. However, numerous attempts to repeat these findings have been unsuccessful, and there is now good reason for thinking that the original finding may have been spurious. Indeed, all the hints of linkage to the major psychoses listed in Table 8.6 must be regarded as extremely tentative.

CANDIDATE GENES

The studies on schizophrenia began with the observation that a partial trisomy of the long arm of chromosome 5 cosegregated with the illness in several affected members. In this way a candidate region of the human genome was selected for more intensive investigation of possible linkage. Obviously an even tighter focus for experimentation can be achieved if, instead of a candidate region, there is a candidate gene available for analysis. Provided that informative polymorphisms can be found in or around the candidate gene, its cosegregation with the disease in question can be put to appropriate testing. This might in the first instance take the form of sibling-pair or affected sibling-pair analysis, but ultimately there will need to be a more comprehensive study of cosegregation in an extended family.

There is no formal definition of what constitutes a candidate gene for any given disorder. Indeed it is often remarked that candidate genes lie in the eye of the beholder, and are no more than inspired or (often) uninspired hunches. This is probably overdismissive. Extensive investigation of the biochemical pathology of many multifactorial disorders has revealed consistent abnormalities in proteins or enzymes, whose encoding genes represent respectable candidates for analysis. This is seen most clearly in attempts to unravel the genetic loci predisposing individuals to premature coronary heart disease and in recent advances in the understanding of Alzheimer's disease.

Coronary heart disease

Cardiovascular disease is the largest single cause of all deaths in developed countries, with about half of these being due to coronary heart disease. The changes in the coronary vessels that precede the formation of atherosclerotic plaques are not well understood, but a working hypothesis suggests that the primary event is damage to the endothelial cells, which form a barrier to the passage of blood constituents into the arterial wall. First-order risk factors for coronary heart disease are hyperlipidaemia, the toxic agents contained in cigarette smoke and mechanical shear induced by hypertension. Less important, but still significant, risk factors are obesity, stress and lack of exercise. Following primary endothelial cell injury, macrophages, monocytes and platelets are attracted by chemotactic substances released and attach to the arterial endothelium and facilitate the formation of the atheromatous plaque. The end event that occludes diseased arteries is thrombus formation of an ulcerated plaque.

Although at first sight coronary heart disease may seem the consequence of a self-indulgent life-style, it has been known for many years that genetic factors are also involved. Twin studies have shown a higher concordance rate in monozygotic compared to dizygotic twins, and this is particularly pronounced when disease occurs before the age of 60 years. Several studies have indicated that having a first-degree relative who has had a myocardial infarction is a more powerful risk predictor than hypercholesterolaemia, cigarette smoking or systolic blood pressure. Estimates of the heritability (a much-abused but quite widely used index of the importance of genetic factors) of ischaemic heart disease are consistently over 50%. There is little doubt that coronary heart disease, for all its obvious clinical heterogeneity, belongs to the class of multifactorial disorders, and that it is

223

Table 8.7. *Mendelian disorders conferring an increased risk of premature coronary heart disease (CHD)*

Disorder	Lipid and/or lipoprotein abnormalities	Risk of CHD
Autosomal recessive		
Lecithin: cholesterol acyltransferase deficiency	All major lipoproteins	Moderate
Hepatic triglyceride lipase deficiency	Hypercholesterolaemia, hypertriglyceridaemia	Moderate
Apolipoprotein AI (apo AI) deficiency	Deficiency of apo AI, low HDL	High
Cerebrotendinous xanthomatosis	Accumulation of bile cholesterol	Moderate
Sisterolaemia	Increased plant sterols in LDL and HDL	High
Autosomal dominant		
Familial combined hyperlipidaemia	Increased apo B, LDL and/or VLDL	High
Familial hypercholesterolaemia	Increased cholesterol and LDL	High

Note: Abbreviations: HDL, LDL and VLDL are high-density, low-density and very low-density lipoproteins.

both legitimate and profitable to approach it by attempting to tease out major susceptibility genes.

As in many other multifactorial disorders, important clues are to be found in Mendelian conditions that confer an increased risk of premature coronary heart disease. The list is quite substantial (Table 8.7). Most of the autosomal recessive conditions are relatively rare. In contrast, the two autosomal dominants in Table 8.7 are amongst the most prevalent of all human monogenic disorders. Sufferers from heterozygous familial hypercholesterolaemia number about 1 in 500 people and 75% of (male) patients have symptoms of coronary heart disease by age 60 years. Even more dramatic is the prevalence of familial combined hyperlipidaemia, estimated at about 0.5% in Western societies and perhaps responsible for 10% of cases of coronary heart disease.

Table 8.8. *Properties of the major plasma apolipoproteins*

Apolipoproteins	% Distribution in				Relative molecular weight	Chromosomal localization
	HDL	LDL	IDL	VLDL		
Apo AI	100				29 000	11q23–q24
Apo AII	100				17 000	1q21–q23
Apo AIV	100				44 000	11q23–qter
Apo B–100		80	10		500 000	2p24–p23
Apo CI	100				6 000	19q13.2
Apo CII	60		10	30	9 000	19q13.2
Apo CIII	60	10	10	20	9 000	11q23–qter
Apo D	100				19 000	3q26.2–qter
Apo E	50				34 000	19q13.2

Note: Abbreviations: as in Table 8.7. IDL, intermediate-density lipoprotein.

The fact that many, but not all, monogenic conditions with predisposition to coronary heart disease involve abnormalities of lipid metabolism suggests that genes affecting the function or quantity of plasma lipids and lipoproteins may be seen as candidate genes. There are four major classes of lipoprotein (Lp) and nine main types of apolipoprotein (apo: see Table 8.8). Each of the nine apolipoprotein genes has been cloned, sequenced and assigned to a specific chromosome. A large part of the work on the molecular genetics of coronary heart disease is concerned with variation in these genes and the contributions of the variation to different types of hypo- and hyperlipidaemia.

In view of its quantitative importance, familial combined hyperlipidaemia (FCHL) is a Mendelian disorder for which documentation of a specific genetic lesion is likely to throw considerable light on the pathogenesis of coronary heart disease. A characteristic feature of FCHL is pleomorphic manifestation of lipid abnormalities even amongst relatives in the same family. About one-third of the patients have hypercholesterolaemia and elevated levels of low-density lipoproteins (LDL), another third have hypertriglyceridaemia and elevated levels of very low-density lipoproteins (VLDL), while the final third show both abnormalities. There is also a striking elevation of levels of apolipoprotein B (apo B), the principal protein consituent of the LDL fraction. However, perhaps surprisingly, linkage analysis in FCHL families has mapped the disorder to the apo AI–CIII–AIV cluster on the long arm of chromosome 11, a triad of genes of very similar genomic structure (Fig. 8.4), which are placed within a 20 kb segment at 11q23–q24, and quite distinct from the apo B locus on 2p24–p23. The relevant gene in the cluster has not yet been identified, but seems unlikely to be apo AI, since mutations at this locus are reported to reduce the levels of high-density lipoprotein (HDL) (Table 8.7). How a putative mutation within this cluster might account for the elevation of levels of apo B in FCHL patients has yet to be explained.

The best understood of the monogenic disorder of lipid metabolism is familial hypercholesterolaemia (FH). Pioneering work by J. Goldstein and M. Brown, who used cultured fibroblasts from rare individuals homozygous for FH, showed the primary biochemical defect to lie in deficient or functionally abnormal cell-surface LDL receptors. This receptor, which is localized in clathrin-coated pits, mediates the removal of cholesterol from plasma by selectively binding the apo B component of the LDL–cholesterolester–apo B complex (Fig. 8.5). After endocytosis of the complex, LDL is degraded by hydrolytic enzymes, the apo B is hydrolysed by proteases, and cholesterolesters hydrolysed by a lysosomal acid hydrolase. Free cholesterol crosses the lysosomal membrane and stabilizes cholesterol concentration by a sophisticated feedback system. Not only does it suppress the rate-controlling enzyme of its own intracellular biosynthesis (HMG–CoA reductase), and the synthesis of further LDL receptors, but it also activates a cholesterol-esterifying enzyme, which permits storage of excess cholesterol as cholesterolesters. Thus the consequences of an inherited defect in LDL receptors is pleotrophic. Most important is the decline in the rate of removal of

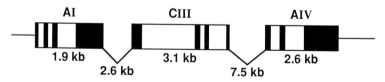

Fig. 8.4. The apo AI–CIII–AIV gene cluster on the long arm of chromosome 16. Exons are shown as filled boxes and introns as open boxes. The sizes of the genes and of the intergenic distances are indicated. From Taylor *et al.* (1987). Copyright © 1987, Ciba Foundation. Reprinted by permission of John Wiley & Sons, Ltd.

plasma LDL, the rise in LDL concentration and the deposition of excess lipid in connective tissue and scavenger cells with the formation of xanthomas and atheromas. FH homozygotes have grossly elevated levels of plasma cholesterol and show frequent signs of coronary heart disease in childhood. In the more common FH heterozygotes, plasma cholesterol levels are elevated approximately twofold and these individuals face a pronounced risk of coronary heart disease in the later years.

The two autosomal dominant conditions FCHL and FH provide useful clues to candidate genes where mutations have a clear role in susceptibility to coronary heart disease. Other genes, where normal variation in structure or controlling elements influences plasma levels of lipoproteins, are likely to be equally or more important in unravelling multifactorial inheritance. One such genetic locus which controls the Lp(a) system is of considerable interest because it provides for the first time a plausible link between the formation of atherosclerotic plaques and the arterial thrombotic events that precipitate heart attacks and strokes. Lp(a) represents a distinct subpopulation of LDL, containing both apo B and a heavily glycosylated protein known as apo(a). Levels of Lp(a) amongst normal individuals range from almost undetectable to more than 1 mg/ml and there is a strong cor-

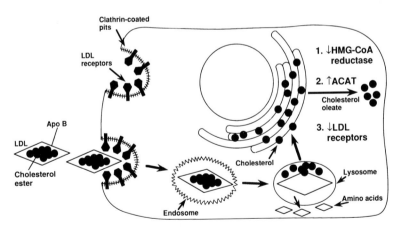

Fig. 8.5. Sequential steps in LDL-receptor-mediated removal of LDL–cholesterolester–apo B complexes from plasma. See the text for details. Feedback control of free cholesterol is exerted through: (1) inhibition of HMG–CoA reductase; (2) stimulation of acyl CoA:cholesterol acyltransferase (ACAT); and (3) reduction in synthesis of further LDL receptors.

relation between high plasma levels and the risk of premature coronary heart disease. To a large extent, levels of Lp(a) are determined genetically, in part by multiple alleles at a single genetic locus that determine the size of apo(a). Smaller apo(a) molecules are associated with elevated Lp(a) plasma concentrations, and vice versa. What makes apo(a) so interesting is its similarity to plasminogen, the precursor of the proteolytic enzyme plasmin, which dissolves fibrin blood clots. Indeed, both apo(a) and plasminogen have been mapped to the same region of chromosome 6 (6q26–q27), and have very similar protein conformations. Lp(a) accumulates on the endothelium of atherosclerotic coronary arteries but not in normal blood vessels. A plausible hypothesis suggests that in individuals with inherited high levels of Lp(a), the molecule is incorporated into damaged endothelial cells and there inhibits the binding of plasminogen and dissolution of the clot by plasmin.

Further evidence for the role of Lp(a) in atherosclerosis comes from a study of plasma concentrations in patients with FH. In this condition, concentrations of Lp(a) in plasma are increased significantly over controls and furthermore are independent of the size of the apo(a) molecule. FH patients with highest levels of Lp(a) have the greatest risk of coronary heart disease. The mechanism of this effect is obscure, but may relate to the excessive burden of plasma LDL, which, in FH patients, interferes with the normal clearance and turnover of Lp(a). However, the fact that two separate genetic loci have been implicated (in this instance) in the risk of coronary heart disease makes the point that gene–gene interactions are likely to be the rule rather than the exception in multifactorial diseases.

This point is reinforced by studies on the genetic variants of apo E. Polymorphism at this locus is controlled by three common alleles specifying distinct isoforms apo E2, apo E3 and apo E4. Apo E2, which differs from the most frequent apo E3 isoform by a single amino acid residue, binds poorly to lipoprotein receptors, and apo E2/ 2 homozygotes might be expected to develop hyperlipidaemia and hypercholesterolaemia. In fact, in the multifactorial condition known as familial type III hyperlipoproteinaemia virtually all patients have the apo E2/2 phenotype. This condition is associated with a high risk of premature coronary heart disease. However, most apo E2/2 homozygotes (perhaps 1% of Western populations) never develop hyperlipidaemia and indeed have subnormal cholesterol levels. Therefore the apo E locus can be only one component of genetic susceptibility and must be modulated by other as yet unidentified genetic and environmental factors.

228

The examples given above suggest that candidate genes conferring susceptibility to coronary heart disease are likely to be many and varied. Apolipoprotein and lipoprotein-receptor genes are in many ways the most obvious and easily investigated sources of variation. In addition some of the autosomal recessive conditions listed in Table 8.7 have their origins in specific deficiencies of enzymes involved in lipoprotein metabolism, e.g. lecithin:cholesterol acyltransferase and hepatic triglyceride lipase deficiencies. But the list of candidate genes is undoubtedly much greater and is currently limited only by the imagination of those who investigate the complex biochemical and cellular pathology of this group of disorders.

Alzheimer's disease
Progressive loss of intellectual capacity, in the form of failing memory and declining ability to make judgements, is one of the almost inevitable consequences of ageing. As the life-span increases, more and more people show clinical signs of dementia, the estimate for the over-85 age group being about 30%. At necropsy, about half of these show the characteristic features of Alzheimer's disease – neuronal loss, senile plaques and neurofibrillary tangles. Clinical diagnosis during the lifetime of the patient is more difficult and usually made by excluding other causes of dementia, the most common of which are those induced by alcholism or by cardiovascular accidents. None the less, it is estimated that up to 5% of over-65s may have Alzheimer's disease.

Given the high and age-dependent frequency of Alzheimer's, it may well be asked whether it is indeed a disease entity rather than an accelerated ageing process. Much of the evidence for the former comes from the study of familial aggregations. Concordance rates in monozygotic twins are about 40%, while the risk to first-degree relatives is of the order of 5% to 10%. While these figures are not particularly impressive, it is clear that in certain families an early-onset form of Alzheimer's disease segregates as an autosomal dominant with high penetrance. Numerous pedigrees of familial Alzheimer's disease (FAD) have now been published, in which the risk to first-degree relatives is very close to 50%. Most of these families are characterized by an age-of-onset in the late 40s or early 50s. Once again, a Mendelian form of what is probably usually a multifactorial disorder has provided a handle for attempts to map a major susceptibility gene.

Investigations of FAD have been assisted enormously by the extensive experience of the pathology of the disorder. The two most characteristic abnormalities of the cortex of patients with Alzheimer's disease are the deposition of intracellular neurofibrillary tangles and of extracellular amyloid plaques. The major protein subunit found both in tangles and in plaques is an insoluble, highly aggregating, small polypeptide with a relative molecular weight of 4500, dubbed amyloid β-protein (or A_4). Determination of the amino acid sequence of amyloid β-protein showed it to be a novel polypeptide of 42 or 43 residues, which had been cleaved from a larger protein, the amyloid precursor protein (APP). The gene encoding APP was cloned and localized to chromosome 21. What made this finding exciting was the prior knowledge that the neurofibrillary tangles and amyloid plaques of Alzheimer's disease are also found in the brains of older patients with Down syndrome. Thus, not only did the APP gene become a prime candidate for a susceptibility gene for FAD, but its chromosomal localization was also known. When several independent investigators mapped the FAD gene to the long arm of chromosome 21, in the region of the APP gene, the conclusion seemed inescapable that the APP gene was a prime susceptibility gene for Alzheimer's disease.

However, perhaps inevitably, the story of Alzheimer's disease is turning out to be a great deal more complicated. In the first place, both the APP and the FAD genes appeared to map outside the 21q22 region commonly associated with triplication in Down syndrome (see Chapter 7), an unexpected finding in view of the common neuro-pathology in both Alzheimer's disease and trisomy 21. Subsequently, several groups showed recombinants between polymorphisms at the APP locus and families in which Alzheimer's disease appeared to be segregating as an autosomal dominant. What was particularly curious about these findings was the fact that FAD appeared to be segregat-ing with chromosome 21 markers. Could there in fact be two separate and distinct chromosome 21 genes conferring susceptibility to Alzheimer's disease?

It now seems reasonably certain that mutation in the APP gene is a major cause of Alzheimer's disease in at least some cases of the disorder. It had been noted previously that in a rare disorder known as hereditary cerebral haemorrhage with amyloidosis of the Dutch type (HCHWA-D), where there is also accumulation of amyloid β-protein in senile plaques, there is a specific mutation in exon 17 of the APP gene. A search for similar mutations in families with early-onset FAD revealed a missense valine-to-isoleucine mutation at position 717 in exon 17 of the APP gene (Fig. 8.6). This particular mutation has been found in several independent early-onset FAD families of different ethnic origins, but not yet in the more common sporadic Alzheimer's disease. Furthermore, careful examination of exons 16 and 17 of the APP gene (the exons that code for the amino acid residues constituting amyloid β-protein; Fig. 8.6) suggests that even in early-onset FAD this type of mutation is a comparatively rare event.

These findings made the point that, in complex disorders of which Alzheimer's disease is a useful model, simple explanations are likely

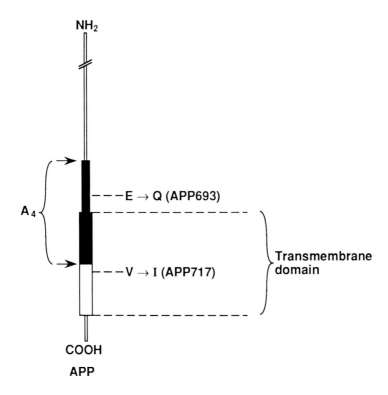

Fig. 8.6. Representation of amyloid β-protein (A_4) and the amyloid precursor protein (APP), from which it is cleaved. Arrows indicate cleavage points in APP, one of which is outside the transmembrane domain and the other within it. The glutamic acid to glutamine change (E→Q) responsible for HCHWA-D (APP693) occurs in an extramembrane region of APP. The valine to isoleucine change in some forms of FAD (APP717) is in the transmembrane region of APP, but probably just outside the A_4 cleavage point.

to be the exception. While there is good evidence that early onset subgroups of FAD map to only chromosome 21 (some obviously to the APP gene and others, perhaps, to another locus at 21q), later onset subgroups have been shown to map to both chromosomes 21 and 19. It is quite possible that three or more genes may be involved in susceptibility, together with gene–gene interactions and the modifying influence of environmental factors. It is possible that mutations similar to those already described for the APP gene in FAD may occur somatically in the ageing brain in sporadic Alzheimer's disease. One must be optimistic that the power of molecular genetic technology in unpicking susceptibility genes locus by locus and exon by exon provides hope that eventually this important disease will be understood more comprehensively.

MUTATION ANALYSIS

In the previous section I discussed how a potential candidate gene for a particular disorder – the example was the APP gene and Alzheimer's disease – could be teased out, initially by segregation analysis and then by the discovery of specific mutations. The ultimate proof that a mutation is causative, rather than coincidentally associated, lies in showing that even if it does not occur in all forms of the disorder it is never found in unaffected individuals. Obviously in some disorders it is tempting to try to skip the laborious and time-consuming linkage analysis of a putative candidate gene and to proceed directly to searching for characteristic sequence changes in that gene. This makes sense if a gene has already been implicated in a disorder by virtue of a characteristic and consistent disease-associated protein pathology. In many of the classical inborn errors of metabolism, which, of course, have the advantage that they show Mendelian modes of transmission, specific enzyme deficiencies have been recognized for many years. In most of these it has not been necessary to demonstrate formally that the gene encoding that particular enzyme segregates with the disorder; instead the investigator can move immediately to cataloguing the range of mutations in the gene.

In multifactorial disorders, the strategy of direct mutation analysis is much less likely to be successful. There are usually far too many candidate genes, each one of which is as likely or as unlikely as the next to be of primary importance, for the investigator to feel it worth while to start using the mutation scanning procedures described in Chapter 3. Some clues are needed that will increase the probability of successful outcome. One useful clue would be if a subset of families with the disorder showed an X-linked mode of inheritance, and if there were a candidate gene on the X chromosome that made more sense of the disorder.

An interesting example of this approach has recently been reported amongst the motor neurone diseases. About 90% of cases of motor neurone disease (or amyotrophic lateral sclerosis) are sporadic and probably multifactorial. The remainder appear to be familial, predominantly with a dominant mode of inheritance. Indeed, random mapping has given clear evidence of linkage in some of these families to a causative gene on the long arm of chromosome 21, very close to the region of the APP gene implicated in familial Alzheimer's disease. However, there is also a subgroup, known as spinal and bulbar muscular atrophy or Kennedy disease, that is obviously X-linked. Not only do males affected with Kennedy disease show the adult-onset muscle weakness and wasting characteristic of most types of motor neurone disease, but they also often have gynecomastia and reduced fertility. This suggested a deficiency in androgen function and focused attention on the androgen-receptor gene, which has been mapped to Xq11–q12. It obviously helped that linkage analysis of Kennedy disease suggested localization in the same region but, all the same, the decision to begin sequence analysis of the androgen-receptor gene in Kennedy disease patients was something of a fishing expedition.

The results were surprising. The androgen-receptor gene has eight exons, seven of which code for protein domains involved in either androgen or DNA binding (Fig. 8.7). However, in Kennedy disease, mutations were found in only the first exon, which encodes a portion of the receptor of unknown function. Furthermore, the type of mutation was most unusual, consisting of a variable amplification of a CAG repeat unit to give an exon about 75 bp larger than usual. CAG codes for glutamine, and normal individuals have a tract of about 20 glutamine residues in this region of their receptor, whereas in Kennedy patients the range is from 40 to 52 glutamine residues. The difference is easy to detect by PCR amplification of the relevant region and inspection of the size of product on an agarose or polyacrylamide gel. No overlap has been seen between normal and affected individuals. A similar type of mutation, though in this case a much larger amplification of a CCG repeat coding for arginine, is a feature of the fragile X syndrome (Chapter 7).

It is not clear why the specific amplification of the CAG repeat in the first exon of the androgen-receptor gene should lead to the degeneration of spinal and bulbar motor neurones in Kennedy

233

disease. Absence of androgen receptors causes one form of testicular feminization, but without muscle weakness. This suggests that the CAG repeat may be involved in tissue-specific regulation of androgen binding. It is also not clear whether some non-Kennedy forms of motor neurone disease might also carry mutations in the androgen-receptor gene. Although this is unlikely, it is probably worth screening sporadic male cases of motor neurone disease, whether or not they show associated gynecomastia, for this particular mutation.

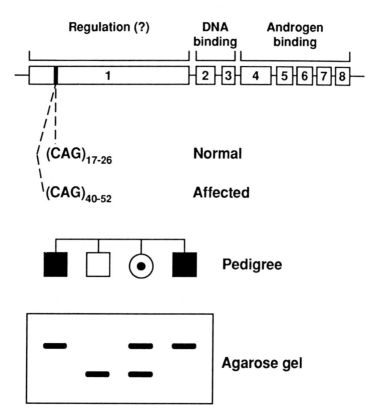

Fig. 8.7. Schematic representation of the androgen-receptor gene showing the eight exons and the domains in the receptor that they control. The CAG amplification-mutation characteristics of Kennedy disease occurs in exon 1. The agarose gel shows the type of patterns seen in a typical pedigree with affected and unaffected male siblings and a carrier female.

SPONGIFORM ENCEPHALOPATHIES

The human spongiform encephalopathies Creutzfeldt–Jacob disease (CJD), Gerstmann–Straussler syndrome (GSS) and kuru are characterized by spongy degeneration of the cerebral grey matter, neuronal loss and proliferation and hypertrophy of astrocytes. They are similar to two transmissible neurodegenerative disorders of animals; scrapie, which occurs in sheep and goats, and bovine spongiform encephalopathy (BSE) or mad cow disease. BSE appears to be the result of the feeding of scrapie-infected sheep offal to cattle, whereas kuru is the consequence of ritualistic cannibalism amongst the tribes of New Guinea. Scrapie and BSE, as well as CJD, GSS and kuru, have all been transmitted to experimental animals by intracerebral innoculation. The infectious agent appears to be an unusual protein, the prion protein (PrP).

Despite evidence for the infectious nature of these conditions, GSS is usually familial, following an autosomal dominant mode of inheritance with reduced penetrance, while some 10% to 15% of cases of CJD are also inherited as autosomal dominants. The extraordinary feature of these diseases (specifically CJD and GSS, and possibly also kuru) is that PrP is encoded by the host chromosomal gene rather than by the infectious prion particle. This distinguishes prions from viruses and also from retroviruses carrying cellular oncogenes. The PrP gene locus is on the short arm of chromosome 20 and consists of a single exon encoding a normal cell-surface glycoprotein found on neuronal cells, lymphocytes and some other tissues. The isoform of the normal prion protein is designated PrP^C. In infected cells a modified isoform PrP^{SC} appears, almost certainly the consequence of post-translational modification. It is not clear how PrP^C is converted to PrP^{SC}, but when PrP^{SC} is introduced from exogenous sources it soon becomes the predominant prion protein, perhaps by a type of chain-reaction catalytic conversion of PrP^C. It now seems very probable that PrP^{SC} is the sole constituent of the infectious prion particle.

A number of characteristic mutations in the PrP gene have been described for familial spongiform encephalopathies (Fig. 8.8). In CJD, there are insertions of octorepeat units at position 53 as well as point mutations at positions 178 and 200. In GSS, point mutations at positions 102, 117 and 198 have been described. Presumably these inherited mutations permit the conversion of PrP^C to PrP^{SC} in appropriate cells.

Even more striking is the recent finding of consistent sequence variation in the PrP genes of sporadic CJD cases. It is known that there is a polymorphism at codon 129 of the gene (Fig. 8.8) with the alternatives of a methionine or a valine residue in PrP^C In the normal population the frequency of the three phenotypes are homozygous methionine 37%, heterozygotes 51% and homozygous valine 12%. However, amongst sporadic cases of CJD there is a large excess of both types of homozygote and hardly any heterozygotes. This was particularly striking in CJD cases where the disease was the result of treatment with contaminated growth hormone and gonadotrophin extracted from pooled batches of cadaveric pituitary glands. Only a small proportion of exposed people contracted CJD; a majority of those who did were homozygous for valine at codon 129 of the PrP gene.

It is thus very probable that the susceptibility gene for CJD and GSS is the PrP gene. In inherited cases, unique mutations in a small set of codons confer a high risk of overt clinical symptoms of neurode-generative disease. In sporadic cases, variation at codon 129 appears to be the primary genetic risk factor. For some patients, contaminated drugs appear to have been the precipitating agents, while in others the exogenous or endogenous factors remain to be discovered.

ANIMAL MODELS

The difficulty in studying multifactorial diseases in humans stems from the imprecision of diagnostic classifications, from clinical and genetic heterogeneity and from variable ages of onset. Studies are also confounded by the paucity of suitable matings between informa-tive couples. One answer is to try to develop animal models in which

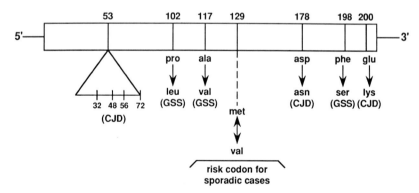

Fig. 8.8. Diagrammatic representation of the PrP gene showing specific mutations responsible for familial CJD and GSS, and the risk codon for sporadic cases.

236

genetic and clinical heterogeneity can be reduced by inbreeding and informative crosses can be carefully designed. The expectation is that some of the same genes that control disease susceptibility in animals will also be found in humans. An important part of this strategy is the construction of human–animal homology maps, so that a gene localized on a specific animal chromosome can by predicted to lie in a particular human chromosomal region.

Documentation of human–animal genetic homologies is now an important part of mapping strategy and forms a substantial component of the regular Human Gene Mapping conferences. Probably the most comprehensive map of a mammalian genome is that of the mouse, and over 500 homologous loci have now been assigned to chromosomes in both human and mouse. Assignments are presented in different formats and include lists of homologous loci in the order of either the 24 human chromosomes or the 21 mouse chromosomes, as well as relative chromosome maps of mouse on human or human on mouse. One convenient system for rapid inspection of regions of homology is the Oxford grid (Fig. 8.9) where the lengths of the vertical and horizontal sides of each rectangle represent the proportionate lengths of human and mouse chromosomes, respectively. The diagram is useful in predicting the location of a human gene when the murine homologue has been mapped, e.g. a candidate human chromosome for a gene mapped to mouse 16 would be 21. The X and Y chromosomes are omitted from the grid, since they are homologous in these two species.

Most of the loci that have been mapped in both systems are for genes encoding enzymes and proteins or for DNA segments. Less progress has been made with disease genes because of the difficulties in correlating a visible mouse phenotype with an analogous human disorder. There is also the problem of differences in the physiology and development of the two species, differences in spontaneous mutation rates and differences in the operation of selective forces. None the less, over 100 loci associated with specific Mendelian conditions in humans have probable or definite homologous conditions in the mouse. Recently the dominantly inherited Waardenberg type I syndrome (wide nose bridge, frontal white blaze of hair, heterochromia iridis and cochlear deafness) was mapped to 2q37 partly on the basis of similarities to the *splotch* mouse mutation previously localized on mouse chromosome 1. Studies on the E1 epileptic mouse have mapped a susceptibility gene to the distal region of chromosome 9, a region showing synteny (correspondence of a series of loci) with human chromosome 3.

An intriguing and innovative approach to mapping susceptibility genes in human multifactorial disorders has emerged from genetic analysis of type I diabetes mellitus in mice. Type I or insulin-dependent diabetes mellitus (IDDM) in humans shows complex inheritance with about 60% of the genetic susceptibility mapping to the HLA class II region (see Fig. 8.1), a result first indicated by sibling-pair analysis. Defining further susceptibility genes has proved extremely difficult. However, there is a murine model, the non-obese diabetic (NOD) mouse, which spontaneously develops IDDM with

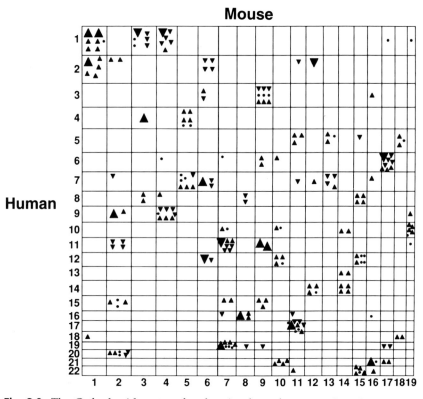

Fig. 8.9. The Oxford grid system for showing homologous regions in human and mouse chromosomes. The sides of the rectangles are proportional to chromosome length. Short arm and long arm assignments are represented by downward and upward pointing triangles, respectively, while unassigned loci are indicated by circles. Large triangles represent at least five loci. From Searle *et al.* (1989).

remarkable similarities to the human disease. In the NOD mouse, a susceptibility gene, *Idd*-1, has also been mapped to the murine major histocompatibility (H-2) complex on chromosome 17. Clearly these animals represent an excellent model system for attempting to locate other relevant IDDM susceptibility genes.

To carry out random linkage analysis of putative susceptibility genes in mice, it was necessary first to develop a set of highly informative markers covering most of the mouse genome. This was achieved by concentrating on microsatellites or CA repeats, which are as well distributed and as polymorphic in mice as they are in humans. By analysis of the association of these markers with disease in experimental crosses between NOD mice and a congenic disease-resistant strain, Todd and colleagues were able to detect two further IDDM susceptibility genes, *Idd*-3 and *Idd*-4. *Idd*-3 mapped to mouse chromosome 3 and *Idd*-4 to mouse chromosome 11, both quite distinct from the *Idd*-1 location on mouse chromosome 17. The most probable human homologous chromosomes are 1 or 4 and 17 (see Fig. 8.9). These remarkable results should stimulate further investigations of relevant human IDDM susceptibility genes by narrowing the region of search to specific chromosomal regions.

SUGGESTED READING

Baron, M. (1991). Genetics of manic depressive illness: current status and evolving concepts. In: McHugh, P. R. and McKusick, V. A. (Editors), *Genes, Brains and Behaviour*, pp. 153–164, Raven Press, New York.

Berg, K. (1987). Genetics of coronary heart disease and its risk factors. In: *Molecular Approaches to Human Polygenic Disease*. Ciba Foundation Symposium 130, pp. 28–33, John Wiley, Chichester.

Cooper, D. N. and Clayton, J. F. (1988). DNA polymorphism and the study of disease associations. *Human Genetics* 78: 299–312.

Cox, N. J. and Spielman, R. S. (1989). The insulin gene and susceptibility to IDDM. *Genetic Epidemiology* 6: 65–69.

Folstein, M. F. and Warren, A. (1991). Genetics of Alzheimer's Disease. In: McHugh, P. R. and McKusick, V. A. (Editors), *Genes, Brains and Behaviour*, pp. 129–136, Raven Press, New York.

Gardiner, R. M. (1990). Genes and epilepsy. *Journal of Medical Genetics* 27: 537–544.

Gelernter, J. and Kidd, K. (1991). The current status of linkage studies in schizophrenia. In: McHugh, P. R. and McKusick, V. A. (Editors), *Genes, Brains and Behaviour*, pp. 137–152, Raven Press, New York.

Glass, I. A. (1991). X-linked mental retardation. *Journal of Medical Genetics* **28**: 361–371.

Goate, A., Chartier-Harlin, M.-C., Mullan, M., Brown, J., Crawford, F., Fidani, L., Giuffra, L., *et al.* (1991). Segregation of a missense mutation in the amyloid precursor protein gene with familial Alzheimer's disease. *Nature (London)* **349**: 704–706.

Goldstein, J. L. and Brown, M. S. (1989). Familial hyper-cholesterolaemia, In: Scriver, C. R., Beaudet, A. L., Sly, W. S. and Valle, D. (Editors), *The Metabolic Basis of Inherited Disease*, 6th Edition, pp. 1215–1250, McGraw-Hill, New York.

Haines, J. L. (1991). Invited editorial: the genetics of Alzheimer disease – a teasing problem. *American Journal of Human Genetics* **48**: 1021–1025.

Humphries, S. E., Talmud, P. J. and Kessling, A. M. (1987). Use of DNA polymorphisms of the apolipoprotein genes to study the role of genetic variation in the determination of serum lipid levels. In: *Molecular Approaches to Human Polygenic Disease*. Ciba Foundation Symposium 130, pp. 128–149, John Wiley, Chichester.

Klein, J., Gutknecht, J. and Fischer, N. (1990). The major histo-compatibility complex and human evolution. *Trends in Genetics* **6**: 7–11.

Kondo, I. and Berg, K. (1990). Inherited quantitative DNA variation in the LPA gene. *Clinical Genetics* **37**: 132–140.

Lander, E. S. and Botstein, D. (1986). Mapping complex genetic traits in humans: new methods using a complete RFLP linkage map. *Cold Spring Harbor Symposia on Quantitative Biology* **51**: 49–62.

La Spada, A. R., Wilson, E. M., Lubahn, D. B., Harding, A. E. and Fishbeck, K. H. (1991). Androgen receptor gene mutations in X-linked spinal and bulbar muscular atrophy. *Nature (London)* **352**: 77–79.

Levy, E., Carman, M. D., Fernandez-Madrid, I. J., Power, M. D., Lieberburg, I., van Duinen, S. G., *et al.* (1990). Mutation of the Alzheimer's disease amyloid gene in hereditary cerebral haemorrhage, Dutch type. *Science* **248**: 1124–1126.

McKusick, V. A. (1990). *Mendelian Inheritance in Man*. 9th Edition, Johns Hopkins University Press, Baltimore, MD.

Ott, J. (1990). Invited editorial: cutting a Gordian knot in the linkage analysis of complex human traits. *American Journal of Human Genetics* **46**: 219–221.

Prusiner, S. B. (1991). Molecular biology of prion diseases. *Science* **252**: 1515–1521.

Rise, M. L., Frankel, W. N., Coffin, J. M. and Seyfried, T. N. (1991). Genes for epilepsy mapped in the mouse. *Science* **253**: 669–673.

Scott, J. (1991). Lipoprotein (a): thrombotic and atherogenic. *British Medical Journal* **303**: 663–664.

Searle, A. G., Peters, J., Lyon, M. F., Hall, J. G., Evans, E. P., Edwards, J. H. and Buckle, V. J. (1989). Chromosome maps of man and mouse. IV. *Annals of Human Genetics* **53**: 89–140.

Siddique, T., Figlewicz, D. A., Pericak-Vance, M. A., Haines, J. L., Rouleau, G., Jeffers, A. J., *et al.* (1991). Linkage of a gene causing familial amyotrophic lateral sclerosis to chromosome 21 and evidence of genetic locus heterogeneity. *New England Journal of Medicine* **324**: 1381–1384.

St. Clair, D., Blackwood, D., Muir, W., Carothers, A., Walker, M., Spowart, G., *et al.* (1990). Association within a family of a balanced autosomal translocation with major mental illness. *Lancet* **336**: 13–16.

Taylor, J. M., Lauer, S., Elshourbagy, N., Reardon, C., Taxman, E., Walker, D., *et al.* (1987). Structure and evolution of human apolipoprotein genes: identification of regulatory elements of the human apolipoprotein E gene In: *Molecular approaches to human polygenic disease*. Ciba Foundation Symposium 130, pp. 70–89, John Wiley, Chichester.

Todd, J. A., Bell, J. I. and McDevitt, H. O. (1987). HLA-DQB gene contributes to susceptibility and resistance to insulin-dependent diabetes mellitus. *Nature (London)* **329**: 599–604.

Todd, J. A., Aitman, T. J., Cornall, R. J., Ghosh, S., Hall, J. R. S., Hearne, C. M., *et al.* (1991). Genetic analysis of autoimmune type I diabetes mellitus in mice. *Nature (London)* **351**: 542–547.

Utermann, G., Hoppichler, F., Dieplinger, H., Seed, M., Thompson, G. and Boerwinkle, E. (1989). Defects in the low density lipoprotein receptor gene affect lipoprotein (a) levels: multiplicative interaction of two gene loci associated with premature atherosclerosis. *Proceedings of the National Academy Sciences, U.S.A.* **86**: 4171–4174.

Weeks, D. E. and Lange, K. (1988). The affected-pedigree member method of linkage analysis. *American Journal of Human Genetics* **42**: 315–326.

Weissmann, C. (1991). A unified theory of prion propagation. *Nature (London)* **352**: 679–683.

Wojciechowski, A. P., Farall, M., Cullen, P., Wilson, T. M. E., Bayliss, J. E., Farren, B., *et al.* (1991). Familial combined hyperlipidaemia linked to the apolipoprotein AI-CIII-AIV gene cluster on chromosome 11q23–q24. *Nature (London)* **349**: 161–164.

9 CURRENT AND FUTURE DEVELOPMENTS

In the previous chapters I have outlined the impact of the new DNA-based technologies on the spectrum of genetic and quasi-genetic diseases. Most of the detail has been concerned with methods of detection of disease-causing and disease-susceptibility genes. In this final chapter I turn to present and future developments in molecular technology and how they are likely to be used in the more practical aspects of clinical management. The first topic – the avoidance of genetic disease – is already a clinical reality, although there is every prospect that new techniques and approaches will make prevention a more formidable part of the geneticist's armentarium. The second topic – gene therapy – remains tantalizingly round the corner. The final topic – the human gene mapping project – is the most exciting prospect of all and likely to influence and illuminate every aspect of medical practice in the latter half of this decade.

AVOIDANCE OF GENETIC DISEASE

Genetic diseases cannot really be cured, since the defective genes are present in all the cells of the body. Most cannot even be managed effectively. There are exceptions, such as the dietary management of phenylketonuria, replacement therapy of factor VIII or IX in the haemophilias, or long-term transfusion for β-thalassaemia. Many of these treatments are both painful and only partly effective. Indeed it can be argued that the use of heart–lung transplantation for patients with end-term cystic fibrosis does little more than increase the burden of the disease for young sufferers and their parents. At present, the only sensible strategy for most genetic diseases is to employ procedures for the avoidance of the occurrence of mutations and their transmission through successive generations.

As shown in Fig. 9.1, avoidance of genetic disease can be visualized as operating at three distinct levels. The first level seeks to identify the origin and specific causes of mutation and to take steps to reduce the frequency. The second level recognizes that many mutations have

242

already occurred in past generations, but that the passage of at least some of these to future generations can be prevented. The third level – the last stand in the avoidance scheme – accepts that fetuses with genetic diseases will inevitably be conceived but offers the option (to those to whom it is morally acceptable) of interrupting the process before the birth of an affected child. Most of those professionally concerned with genetic diseases would accept that level 1 avoidance is the most desirable strategy on ethical, social and economic grounds. At present, however, level 3 avoidance through prenatal diagnosis and screening is proving the most effective option.

AVOIDANCE OF MUTATION

A distinction must be made between germ-line mutations, which damage oocytes or sperm before fertilization and which will be present in the DNA of all the cells of the developing zygote, and somatic mutations, which affect a more limited set of cells and organs

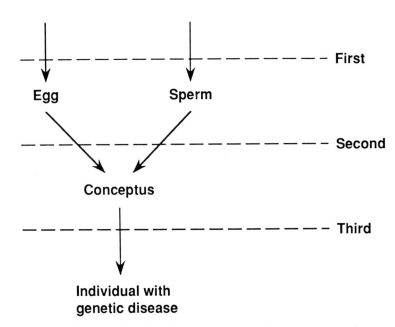

Fig. 9.1. Three levels of avoidance of genetic disease.

243

at some stage of the growth of the embryo. The latter is often referred to as teratogenesis. In some respects the difference may seem artificial. A child with retinoblastoma may have a germ-line mutation and a somatic mutation in retinal cells or two somatic mutations in only retinal cells; in both cases a cancer of the eye results. But in other respects the difference is crucial. Somatic mutations are not transmitted to the progeny of affected individuals whereas germ-line mutations can be and often are. Furthermore, a germ-line mutation can render an individual susceptible to further somatic mutations in a range of tissues and organs, something we have already noted with respect to the retinoblastoma and p53 genes (Chapter 6). It is no surprise, therefore, that society has become increasingly determined to protect young men and women from potential mutagenic effects.

A major problem in avoiding mutation is that we are still largely ignorant of the sources and mechanisms of mutagenic agents in humans. This may seem a surprising statement in view of frequently expressed concerns about the damaging effects of ionizing radiation and the obvious fears about the genetic consequences of accidents such as those at the nuclear reactors at Three Mile Island and Chernobyl. There is no doubt that irradiating mice and other experimental animals with X-rays or γ-radiation induces both chromosome aberrations and gene mutations; the difficulty lies in extrapolating the data to human populations. The largest human 'experiment' to be studied intensively, the consequence of dropping atomic bombs on Hiroshima and Nagasaki, has revealed no definitive evidence of higher incidences of genetic abnormalities in survivors' offspring than in a control unexposed population. Studies on the children of parents who have received pelvic radiotherapy and on the children of radiologists have also been inconclusive. None the less, there is an obvious worry that a hidden load of serious recessive mutations may take many generations to be revealed. It thus makes good sense to avoid exposure to all unnecessary radiation and particularly to gonadal irradiation in those who have yet to conceive. Unfortunately, it is not possible to avoid natural radiation, and this constitutes a high proportion of the total load in most human populations (Table 9.1).

Other potential sources of mutation are environmental chemicals, medically prescribed drugs and common viruses. In those that have been adequately studied, the effects are predominantly teratogenic and therefore presumably somatic. The identification of a fetal alcohol syndrome has pinpointed the dangers of even quite modest intake of alcohol during pregnancy. The thalidomide disaster highlighted the

Table 9.1. *Average radiation load of human populations*

Source	Dose (mrem/year)
Natural background	
Cosmic radiation	~ 50
Terrestrial radiation	~ 60
Ingestion of radioactive elements	~ 20
	130
Avoidable radiation	
Medical diagnostics	~ 50
Atomic-bomb fallout	~ 8
Minor sources	~ 2
	60

Source: Vogel and Motulsky (1986).

need for closer inspection of the potential teratogenic effects of relatively well-known drugs. Congenital malformations associated with rubella infection are well recognized and now largely avoided by systematic immunization. The difficulty with all these teratogens is that each needs to be evaluated separately and there are few rules suitable for general extrapolation.

One major source of genome mutations, and perhaps the single most common origin of congenital abnormality, is maternal age. The increased risk of bearing a child with Down syndrome (trisomy 21) in older mothers has been known for many years, while more recently it has become apparent that there is also a maternal age dependence for trisomies 13 and 18, for Klinefelter syndrome and for the 47,XXX syndrome. The risk of a major chromosome abnormality in the fetus rises almost exponentially after maternal age 35. Older mothers can undergo prenatal karyotype diagnosis in either the first or the second trimesters and in this way protect themselves from the birth of an affected child (level 3 avoidance). But far less attention has been paid to a level 1 avoidance strategy – persuading women to have their babies in their early- and mid-20s when they are biologically most suited to childbirth. For obvious reasons this is currently deemed socially and economically unacceptable. In many developed countries there has been a pronounced trend to later childbearing in recent years. This is shown in the data for England and Wales in Fig. 9.2. The application of widespread prenatal diagnosis can prevent the birth of many of these chromosomally abnormal babies, but for a variety of reasons (social, organizational and ethical) the take-up of a prenatal diagnosis option by the older mother has always been patchy and far from complete.

AVOIDANCE OF TRANSMISSION OF MUTATIONS
With the exception of severe early-onset autosomal dominants and a few X-linked recessives, where new mutations predominate, most genetic diseases are the result of mutations that have occurred many generations in the past. Although the mutations themselves cannot be avoided, in theory their transmission to future generations can. Unfortunately, in most cases this means forgoing reproduction. Many genetic centres now operate registers and collect extended pedigrees of families in which serious autosomal dominant and X-linked recessive disorders are segregating. The purpose of such registers is to flag young people at or near reproductive age so that they may be counselled and advised of their risks of passing mutant genes to their offspring. Autosomal dominant conditions with late age of onset and low mutation rates are particularly well suited to registration, since it is often possible to collect a majority of cases into a small

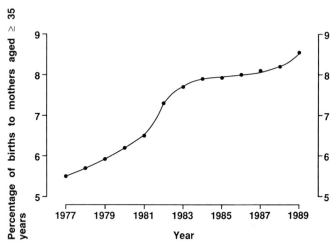

Fig. 9.2. The increasing trend to later childbirth in England and Wales, 1977–89. Adapted from *Birth Statistics*, Office of Population and Census Surveys, HMSO, 1989.

set of extended families. An example of a large Huntington's disease pedigree is shown in Fig. 9.3. It is obvious that large numbers of individuals have substantial risks of inheriting this appalling disease and passing it on to their children. At the very least they should be aware of this fact, and free to make informed decisions about reproduction. In practice, very few couples with a major risk of passing a crippling disease on to their offspring are prepared to forgo reproduction. Indeed, until the advent of prenatal diagnosis, genetic counselling of such families was a frustrating and largely ineffective exercise.

PRENATAL DIAGNOSIS

As suggested earlier, prenatal diagnosis, followed by selective termination of pregnancy, is currently the most effective way of avoiding genetic diseases. It is also the most controversial. Many

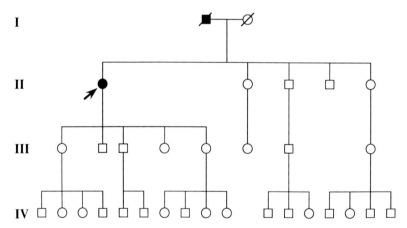

Fig. 9.3. A typical Huntington's disease pedigree. At the time of ascertainment of the proband (arrowed), who had an affected father, there were four siblings in generation II with 50% risk, eight individuals in generation III with 25% risk, and 17 individuals in generation IV at 12.5% risk. None was aware of the risk, since the diagnosis in the affected individual in generation I had been kept secret. Only the use of genetic registers can help to prevent the relentless transmission of this disease. Squares represent male individuals; circles represent females. Open symbols represent individuals of unaffected or undetermined status; filled symbols represent affected individuals. Symbols that are scored through represent deceased individuals.

247

doctors, trained to value life and to try to preserve it at almost any cost, find the concept of abortion repugnant. It does not help to call it therapeutic abortion, a practice in many genetic centres in the U.S.A. Most couples at risk of conceiving a child with a serious genetic disease are appalled that their only realistic reproductive option is to take the chance that a pregnancy may have to be interrupted. Much has been written about the ethics of aborting genetically defective fetuses and fears have been expressed that this may devalue our attitudes to the mentally and physically handicapped. There is little point in rehearsing these debates except to say that the gulf between pro-life and pro-choice groups seems, if anything, to be widening. The medical profession as a whole has reluctantly accepted that prenatal diagnosis is the least bad of a set of unhappy options. This is undoubtedly influenced by the finding that some couples, who initially refuse to accept the concept of abortion, do so when they find that their fetus is affected.

Prenatal diagnosis began slowly in the late 1960s, when it was noted that amniotic-fluid cells were fetal in origin and therefore able to provide information on the genotype of the unborn child. Initially it was concerned with chromosomal abnormalities, then with inborn errors of metabolism defined by defective enzymes and proteins, and slightly later with congenital malformations such as neural-tube defects diagnosed by levels of alphafetoprotein in amniotic fluid. By the mid 1970s, most genetic centres were monitoring high-risk pregnancies for these three classes of genetic and quasi-genetic disease.

The advent of molecular genetic techniques has had a major impact on prenatal diagnosis, and especially on the diagnosis of Mendelian disorders. Several factors contributed to this advance. The technical ability to sample the trophoblast by chorionic-villus biopsy shifted prenatal diagnosis from the second to the first trimester of pregnancy and made it more acceptable to mothers who disliked the idea of aborting a fetus whose movements had already been felt. Chorionic-villus biopsy by either transcervical or transabdominal routes provides a sample that is rich in DNA and particularly appropriate for both direct and indirect gene tracking. Mendelian disorders, in which the relevant gene is not expressed amongst the limited protein and enzyme repertoire of cultured amniotic fluid cells (e.g. haemophilias, haemoglobinopathies, phenylketonuria), could now be diagnosed by DNA techniques. Other Mendelian disorders, in which the defective gene had yet to be cloned and characterized (e.g. Huntington's disease) could be tracked by the indirect linkage methods outlined in Chapter 5. It is reasonable to expect that within a few years most

Table 9.2. *Summary of prenatal diagnosis by DNA-based methods carried out in Scotland between 1987 and 1991*

Disorder	1987	1988	1989	1990	1991	All years
α_1-Antitrypsin deficiency			8	6	5	19
Alport syndrome					1	1
Androgen insensitivity					1	1
β-Thalassaemia					1	1
Choroideraemia	1	2	1	0	4	8
Cystic fibrosis	10	12	13	23	20	78
Haemophilia A	2	1	1	0	1	5
Hereditary neuropathies				1	1	2
Huntington's disease		2	9	5	10	26
Myotonic dystrophy				1	1	2
Ornithine transcarbamylase deficiency					2	2
Retinitis pigmentosa	1	2	2	2	3	10
Sickle cell anaemia					1	1
Spinal muscular atrophy					1	1
von Willebrand disease					1	1
X-linked muscular dystrophy	4	5	12	8	13	42
Total						200

single-genetic-locus defects will become amenable to prenatal diagnosis by these methods.

One of the responses to the new DNA technology has been the emergence of molecular genetic diagnostic laboratories offering a range of prenatal and carrier-detection service options. An indication of the workload of the Scottish laboratory consortium is shown in Table 9.2. To some extent the workload reflects the ethnic make-up of the population (e.g. very little demand for prenatal diagnosis of haemoglobinopathies) and in other respects it marks doctors' enthusiasms and perceptions of the likely burden of a genetic disorder (e.g. no demand for prenatal diagnosis of phenylketonuria). Most requests have been made for prenatal diagnosis and carrier detection of cystic fibrosis and the X-linked muscular dystrophies, neither of which disorders can be tackled by any other than DNA diagnostic techniques. Now that the fragile X gene has been cloned, it may be expected that the demand for prenatal diagnosis and carrier detection in this disorder will greatly increase.

An unusual form of prenatal diagnosis has been devised and applied to Huntington's disease. This is a late-onset autosomal dominant with particularly distressing mental and physical symptoms. Although the Huntington's gene has not (at the time of writing) been cloned, DNA markers have been available since 1983 for indirect tracking in families in which it segregates (Chapter 5). This has been the basis for a presymptomatic test on high-risk individuals who might or might not have inherited the gene from an affected parent. However, telling a high-risk person that he or she carries the Huntington's gene is in effect a delayed death sentence, for that person now knows that all the awful consequences of the

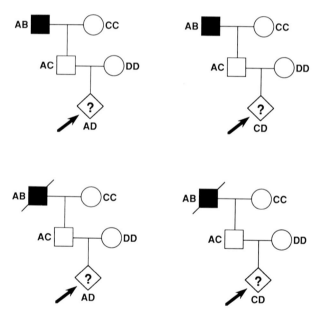

Fig. 9.4. Prenatal-exclusion testing for Huntington's disease using polymorphic DNA markers tightly linked to the disease locus. In each of the four pedigrees illustrated, it is possible to conclude that the fetus, if it has inherited markers AD, has the same 50% risk as its father (markers AC) or, if it has inherited markers CD, that it has not inherited a risk chromosome from the affected grandparent. A diamond represents a fetus. See Fig. 9.3 for explanation of other symbols.

disease will inevitably occur, and there is no management or treatment of the disorder. Many high-risk individuals cannot face this prospect, and yet wish to have their own children without passing on the gene.

Using linked DNA markers it is possible to carry out an incomplete type of prenatal diagnosis of Huntington's disease, called prenatal-exclusion testing. This is illustrated in Fig. 9.4. It is possible to exclude passage of the Huntington's gene in 50% of pregnancies. In the other 50%, transmission cannot be excluded and parents usually opt for termination of pregnancy. The important feature of prenatal-exclusion testing is that the risk status of the parent remains unchanged; no attempt is made to ascertain whether or not he or she carries the Huntington's gene. With luck, these parents can have children whose chance of inheriting the mutant gene is effectively excluded.

PREIMPLANTATION DIAGNOSIS
A development that is already scientifically possible, but as yet of unproven safety and efficacy, is to analyse the genetic status of the morula-stage embryo prior to artificial implantation. Two general procedures are available for gaining access to suitable embryos. In one, fertilization takes place in vivo, either by natural coitus or by artificial insemination, and blastocysts are then flushed from the uterine cavity by gentle lavage. In the other, ovulation is stimulated in the woman, eggs recovered from the ovary by laparoscopy, and the recovered eggs fertilized in vitro and cultured to the four- to eight-cell stage (Fig. 9.5). The former method – in vivo fertilization – has the advantage that diagnostic procedures are carried out on later blastocysts with up to 100 cells, and the biopsied sample is of extra-embryonic trophoectoderm. However, there is a great deal more experience of in vitro fertilization and much of the early human experimentation has been on such four- to eight-cell embryos.

In principle, it is possible to test blastocysts for the presence of genetic abnormalities by either non-invasive or invasive procedures. Non-invasive procedures are necessarily indirect and seek to analyse the release of proteins, enzymes, growth factors or metabolites into the medium in which the blastocyst is cultured. They are limited by the availability of suitable micro-assays and, more important, by the fact that many diagnostically significant genes are probably not transcribed at such an early stage of development. In fact it is very doubtful that non-invasive techniques will make a significant contribution to preimplantation diagnosis. At present there is little alternative but to biopsy the blastocyst for diagnostic purposes and then to implant

251

the remaining cell mass in the hope that its integrity has not been compromised.

In such invasive procedures it is absolutely necessary to be able to detect abnormalities in only one or two cells detached from the blastocyst. This effectively rules out conventional karyotype analysis. It is, however, possible to use in situ hybridization with chromosome-specific probes that target reiterated sequences characteristic of particular chromosomes. Such methods are likely to become available for chromosome 21 and might well be used for screening women at risk for Down syndrome. They have already been used to detect the presence of a Y chromosome, and may have value in sexing blastocysts in women who are carriers of serious X-linked recessive disorders, and who may wish to avoid the implantation of an XY embryo.

It is probable that preimplantation diagnosis will be applied initially to Mendelian disorders in which specific gene mutations are detected by PCR-mediated techniques. The amplification power of the PCR

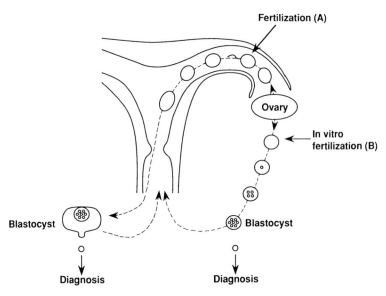

Fig. 9.5. The two routes for preimplantation diagnosis. A. After natural or artificial in vivo fertilization, the blastocyst is flushed from the uterine cavity and a cell removed for diagnosis. B. An egg is recovered from the ovary, fertilized in vitro, and the blastocyst grown to the eight-cell stage prior to diagnosis. In each case, genetically normal blastocysts would be re-implanted.

(and especially the nested variation: Chapter 3) is such that specific DNA sequences in single cells can be visualized quite readily as discrete bands on analytical gels. Preliminary experiments have shown that it is technically possible to detect gene deletions in Duchenne muscular dystrophy, the ΔF_{508} allele in cystic fibrosis and the β^s allele in sickle cell anaemia. However, there are still unresolved problems to be confronted before preimplantation diagnosis becomes a clinical reality. One of these is the development of rigorous containment facilities, which will be necessary to avoid accidental contamination, by extraneous cells or DNA, of the single cell on which the analysis is being carried out. Another more important problem is whether the removal of a cell from a four- to six-cell blastocyst reduces the success rate of the subsequent pregnancy or leads to unrelated abnormalities in the fetus. Some early experiments, in which a single cell was removed for sexing, suggest that a pregnancy success rate of about 35% per implanted embryo can be expected. This is somewhat better than the pregnancy success rate achieved for in vitro fertilization management of infertility.

An alternative to preimplantation diagnosis, and one that avoids the ethical problem of destroying genetically defective blastocysts, is polar-body analysis. The first polar body is the discarded product of the first meiotic division in the oocyte and thus contains the genetic material that will not form part of the embryo. In a female who is heterozygous for a recessive disorder, the presence of a mutation in the polar body signals a normal gene in the secondary oocyte, and vice versa. However, if recombination has occurred during meiotic prophase, both the polar body and the secondary oocyte will be 'heterozygous' for the mutation (Fig. 9.6). Thus, polar-body analysis seeks 'homozygosity' for the mutation in question and uses the corresponding secondary oocyte for fertilization and implantation. No direct tests are actually carried out on the implanted material, and the analysed polar bodies are Nature's discards.

PRENATAL SCREENING

As a means of ensuring that high-risk couples avoid the birth of an affected child, prenatal diagnosis has been a source of reassurance to many anxious parents. But as a means of reducing birth prevalence of serious genetic disorders it is not particularly effective. The reason for this is that indication of risk is often based on the existence of an affected child, and thus prenatal diagnosis seeks to prevent recurrence rather than occurrence. In theory, only one in four children with autosomal or X-linked recessive conditions are recurrences, while the majority represent the first indication that the one or both parents are carriers of mutant genes. More than 95% of children with neural-tube defects are born to parents who have nothing in their family history to alert the parents or doctors to the possibility of such distressing outcome. Even though older mothers are a recognized risk category for bearing children with chromosome anomalies, offering prenatal diagnosis to all who are 35 or older will reduce the birth prevalence of Down syndrome by only about 35%.

The answer to this problem lies in devising forms of prenatal screening that can be applied to whole populations or the whole of particular ethnic subgroups. Screening is still a relatively contentious issue, in that it changes the relationship between doctor and patient. In conventional medical practice, the patient initiates the consultation and seeks the benefit of the doctor's experience and advice. There is an implied contract based on the concept that the doctor will do no

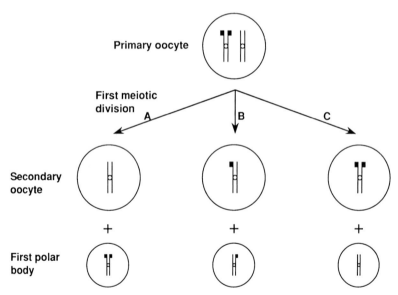

Fig. 9.6. Prenatal diagnosis of polar-body analysis. The primary oocyte is from a mother heterozygous for an autosomal recessive mutation, with the mutation marked as a filled square. In A and C, there has been no recombination during the first meiotic division, whereas in B recombination has occurred. Since the polar body in A is 'homozygous' for the mutation, the corresponding oocyte is 'homozygous' normal and can be used for fertilization and implantation.

harm. By contrast, in all forms of screening the first step is taken by the doctor or medical authority, who invites a general group to undergo a procedure that will be of direct benefit to only a minority. There may well be some consequential harm to a few. It is obviously important that screening programmes be designed to maximize benefit and to minimize harm. This is particularly true in prenatal screening, where the end result could be termination of pregnancy.

The first large-scale screening programme was initiated in the U.K. in the late 1970s. It was founded in the observation that mothers carrying fetuses with neural-tube defects (anencephaly and spina bifida) tended to have elevated levels of maternal-serum alpha-fetoprotein (AFP). Maternal-serum AFP screening has been highly effective in reducing the birth incidence of these serious disorders and is now quite widely available in Europe and the U.S.A. Subsequently it was found that mothers carrying fetuses with Down syndrome had lower than normal levels of serum AFP, lower than normal levels of unconjugated oestriol and higher than normal levels of human chorionic gonadotrophin. This triple biochemical test, combined with assessment of the age-specific risk, is now being used to screen more extensively for fetal Down syndrome, and promises to raise the proportions of cases detectable to between 60% and 70%.

Both neural-tube defect and Down syndrome screening programmes use biochemical measurements of risk and are focused on the mother alone. More germane to the molecular genetic age are programmes directed at Mendelian autosomal recessives, in which the primary objective is the detection of couples where both mother and father are heterozygotes. Normally, heterozygous status is revealed only when a couple has an affected child. But obviously if heterozygote couples could be identified in advance of such an event, the birth incidence of serious autosomal recessive disorders could be reduced substantially. This has, in fact, been achieved both for Tay–Sachs disease and for β-thalassaemia, in the former case using levels of serum hexosaminidase A and in the latter case size and haemoglobin content of red blood cells as primary indicators of parental heterozygosity.

The most exciting programme of prenatal screening for a Mendelian disorder, and one which may well be a prototype for the future, is that directed at cystic fibrosis (CF). It is the first to rely entirely on molecular genetic techniques, both for heterozygote detection and prenatal diagnosis, and therefore the first that has had to grapple with the problem of genetic heterogeneity. In Tay–Sachs disease, heterozygotes have half-normal activities of serum hexosaminidase A, and doubtful cases can be resolved by assay of white blood cell enzyme. In β-thalassaemia, heterozygotes have abnormal red blood cell indices and elevated levels of Hb A_2. But in CF the encoded product of the gene responsible, cystic fibrosis transmembrane conductance regulator (CFTR), is expressed in only a limited range of epithelial cells that are not easily accessible to sampling. The only answer is to search for mutations in genomic DNA, which can of course be obtained from any nucleated cell.

The range of different mutations in the CFTR gene is now extensive, with over 150 described. As shown in Fig. 9.7 they are found in virtually every one of the 27 exons, as well as including a number of splice-site mutations at the beginnings and ends of the introns. Attempting to search for the presence of each one of these mutations on a population-wide basis is economically impossible with current technology. Any screening programme must therefore make the difficult decision to limit the search to the most prevalent alleles in the local population and accept the fact that some carriers will inevitably be missed.

Because CF is a serious life-shortening disease (current median survival to early- or mid-20s), it has been felt worthwhile instituting

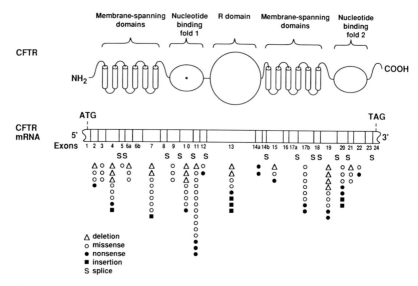

Fig. 9.7. The spectrum of mutations found in the CFTR gene. The diagram shows the 27 exons in CFTR mRNA and the approximate positions of some 110 mutations. A schematic representation of the CFTR protein is shown at the top.

256

pilot trials of heterozygote screening in Caucasian populations where the incidence is high. There has been some argument about where to target such screening. In theory, identification of heterozygotes prior to reproduction allows options of changing partners, undergoing artificial insemination by a screened donor (for a heterozygous woman), or foregoing having children. In practice, these options are unlikely to be acted on, as evidenced by experience with Tay–Sachs disease and β-thalassaemia. It therefore makes sense to carry out screening as close to reproduction as possible and perhaps even during pregnancy. Pregnant women have a heightened awareness of their chances of bearing affected infants and are usually willing to take whatever steps are offered to avoid this happening. Pregnancy is often a convenient turnstile for providing screening on an equitable basis.

Two different types of prenatal screeing for CF are now being offered on a trial basis to U.K. populations. One model uses a two-step approach; pregnant women are offered testing for a set of CFTR mutations, and if found to be negative are reassured that their pregnancy has a low residual risk (Fig. 9.8). If a mutation is identified, the woman's partner is then tested for the same (or perhaps a larger set of) alleles. Couples in which both the man and the woman have identified mutations have a one in four risk of an affected infant and usually opt for prenatal diagnosis. The weakness in this scheme occurs with couples when the woman is positive and her partner negative, for the residual risk of adverse outcome is still fairly high. There are no effective practical steps that can be taken to reduce this residual risk, and there is some concern that undue anxiety may be generated in such positive–negative couples.

An alternative model has been termed couple screening. The unit of risk is the couple, and they are advised of their high-risk status only when mutations are identified in both partners. All other couples – including those where both partners are negative, where only one partner is tested and found to be negative, or where one partner is positive and the other negative – are treated as low risk, and given a composite figure for the chance of having a CF-affected child (Fig. 9.9). This type of couple screening has the virtue of avoiding the need for detailed genetic counselling necessary in two-step screening, and should spare undue anxiety in all but the small proportion of one in four risk cases. Whether it is a practical method of population screening is yet to be discovered.

One question that has been raised by the recently initiated trials of CF screening is whether this represents a Pandora's box. Will pregnancy become a time in a woman's life when she is bombarded with information on risks of a range of genetic diseases in her unborn child, and when she may have difficult decisions to make about a whole series of offered tests for heterozygosity? There is no doubt that the new genetic technologies are providing the ability to screen for more and more Mendelian disorders, and there is equally obviously a danger that the enthusiasm of screeners will lead to the introduction of excessive and inappropriate testing. This is not a situation where one can reasonably expect the lay person to make judgements on issues such as the likely severity and burden of the particular disorder or the protective value of a heterozygote test. The

Two-step screening

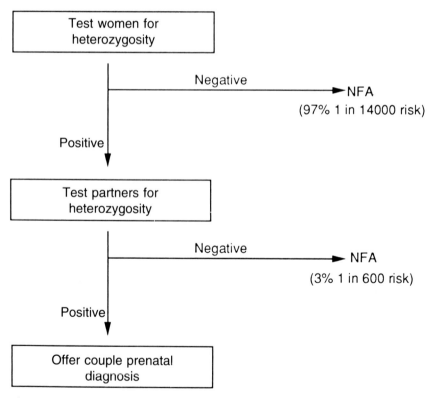

Fig. 9.8. Model of two-step prenatal screening for CF. Estimates of risk are based on the ability to detect 83% of CF alleles. NFA, no further action taken.

responsibility falls instead on the medical profession as a whole. Only they have the necessary detailed knowledge to give approval to prospective new types of screening. Although this is not a particularly fashionable view in an era that calls for more lay involvement in medical decision-making, it is grounded in the reality that a very large majority of patients still look to their doctors for guidance in selecting options set before them. The implied contract between doctor and patient, characteristic of more traditional medical care, also holds for screening. The person offered screening is entitled to assume that any suggested procedure has been carefully assessed and considered by his or her medical practitioner, and that the fact that it is offered at all carries an implied stamp of approval.

Couple screening

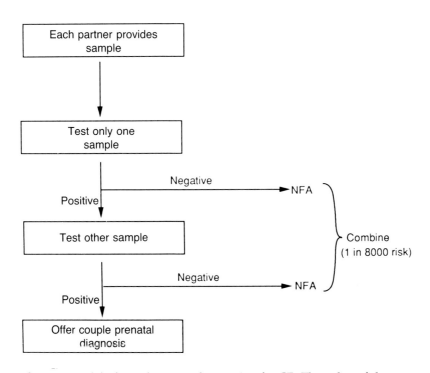

Fig. 9.9. Model of couple prenatal screening for CF. The value of the combined-risk estimate is based on the ability to detect 83% of mutant CF alleles. NFA, no further action taken.

Within this context it is worth considering whether there are other Mendelian conditions that might be suitable candidates for widescale heterozygote testing. Amongst the serious autosomal recessive disorders, the haemoglobinopathies (α- and β-thalassaemias, sickle cell anaemia), Tay–Sachs disease and CF all have relatively high incidences in different ethnic groups and are already the subject of trial screening programmes. It is difficult to envisage any other autosomal recessive with the right combination of severity, poor treatability and high incidence being added to this list in the near future. The relatively common and severe X-linked recessives, such as Duchenne muscular dystrophy and haemophilia A, are characterized by a high rate of new mutations, which would make prenatal screening relatively ineffective. Perhaps the most likely candidate is the fragile X syndrome (Chapter 7). Not only is it the most common source of inherited mental handicap (1 in 1500 males, 1 in 2000 females), but all mothers of affected boys have a premutation, which can now be detected by a relatively simple PCR amplification of the CGG repeat region at Xq27.3. There are special counselling problems associated with the peculiar inheritance of the full-blown syndrome (Chapter 7), but in terms of incidence, severity and lack of any form of treatment it is obviously a condition for which prenatal screening must be seriously considered.

GENE THERAPY

The very poor prognosis for many children born with genetic diseases, and the fact that avoidance strategies are most effective at the ethically dubious level of termination of pregnancy, have continued to prompt a search for more effective methods of management and treatment. Ultimately the goal must be one of curing the disease by directing treatment to the molecular site of the defect – the mutant gene itself – rather than to the biochemical and cellular consequences of mutant gene products. Advances in the understanding of the function and control of genes, together with the existence of over 1000 cloned human genes, are now beginning to make the eventual prospect of gene therapy one worth seriously pursuing. Indeed, a new journal *Human Gene Therapy*, devoted to this topic, was launched in 1990. None the less, the technical and ethical obstacles to bringing gene therapy into clinical practice remain formidable, and real progress is likely to be slow.

It is possible in principle to conceive of two rather different approaches to gene therapy (Table 9.3). Normal genes could be introduced into the germ line with the objective of eliminating or prevent-

Table 9.3. *Principles of gene therapy*

Germ-line gene therapy	Introduction of normal gene into germ line in order to eliminate or prevent expression of a mutant gene 'Corrective gene therapy'
Somatic gene therapy	Introduction of normal gene into somatic cells in order to augment or replace the product of the mutant gene 'Augmentation or replacement therapy'

ing the expression of a mutant gene. It is the method of choice for dominantly inherited disorders, where, by definition, the product of a single mutant gene is sufficient to cause biochemical or cellular damage. Some form of recombination between inserted normal and endogenous mutant genes would be required. It is a bold approach in that corrected genes would remain (at least in theory) corrected in the offspring of the recipient. However, uncertainties about the exact consequences of gene insertion make it dangerous to contemplate a strategy that would perpetuate altered or new genes in future generations. Although germ-line gene therapy is being actively pursued in experimental animal models, it is, for the present, ruled out as an approach to human genetic diseases.

In somatic gene therapy the objective is to introduce a normal gene into an appropriate tissue in such a way that it would either replace or augment the product of the defective gene. There is no need to remove the mutant DNA sequence, and the correction would be limited, tissue-restricted and not passed to the offspring of the recipient. In ethical terms it is little different to blood transfusion or organ transplantation. Replacement or augmentation gene therapy is particularly suitable for those autosomal or X-linked recessive disorders in which mutation has resulted in a profound depletion or complete absence of the encoded protein product. It would probably be sufficient if the inserted gene produced enough product to convert the recipient to, in effect, a heterozygous phenotype; indeed in many disorders there is evidence that comparatively low levels of the normal protein product would suffice.

Although the goals of replacement gene therapy seem comparatively simple, the difficulties in bringing this technique to successful fruition are daunting. These include finding an appropriate tissue to target, devising means of transfecting DNA into recipient cells, ensuring that the transfected DNA is both integrated stably and expressed stably and appropriately, and avoiding the disruption of normal genes and the activation of inappropriate genes. Finally, the candidate disorder should be a serious one for which no other form of treatment is effective, and based on a mutation that has been well characterized at the gene and protein level.

RECIPIENT CELLS

The initial focus for disorders suitable for gene therapy were those where the defect was expressed primarily in cells of haematopoietic lineage. Bone marrow cells can be sampled quite easily, manipulated in culture for DNA transfection and returned to the recipient. However, the vast majority of recognizable blood cell precursors are already terminally differentiated and survive in the circulation for only a limited time before they are destroyed. Stem cells, the self-sustaining precursor cell populations, would have to be the targets for transfection. Human stem cells cannot easily be recognized and optimistic guesses suggest that their fractional concentration may be as low as 10^{-3} to 10^{-5} of the total. Either transfection would have to be extremely efficient or transfected cells would have to have a selective advantage over non-transfected cells to achieve any degree of replacement of protein product. Experiments in mice show that while it is possible to transfect authentic stem cells using a retroviral vector, expression of the transfected genes tends to be transient and unstable.

An alternative strategy is to view gene therapy as an on-going process of treatment rather than a once-and-for-all cure. This is the thinking behind current attempts to treat children who suffer from severe combined immunodeficiency due to a profound defect in adenosine deaminase (ADA) activity. The ADA gene can be inserted quite efficiently into T-lymphocytes using a retroviral vector and these cells can be cultured in vitro using interleukin-2 as a growth stimulant. Transfected T-lymphocytes from ADA-deficient patients produce relatively high levels of enzyme in culture. The plan is to transfuse the patients with ADA-bearing lymphocytes in the hope that enough enzyme would be produced to reverse the consequences of the immunodeficiency. Since T-cells are relatively short lived, such treatment would have to be repeated.

There is similar thinking behind plans to recruit another disorder, CF, to the gene-therapy stable. The main source of morbidity in CF is the progressive lung damage, which follows colonization by

Table 9.4. *Potential delivery systems for gene therapy*

Chemical	Calcium phosphate microprecipitates
	DEAE–dextran
	Dimethylsulphoxide
Cell fusion	Microcell fusion
	Protoplast fusion
Physical	Microinjection
	Electroporation
	Laser micropuncture
Viral	Retroviruses
	Adenoviruses
	Adeno-associated viruses

Pseudomonas aeruginosa and other micro-organisms. It is presumed, though it has not been established definitively, that this is due to the secretion of an abnormal mucus into the airways as a result of defective functioning of the cystic fibrosis transmembrane conductance regulator (CFTR). Of course, airway epithelium can not be removed, treated and replaced, but it can be reached comparatively easily by inhaler-propelled aerosols. If the CFTR gene or CFTR cDNA could be integrated into a suitable vector, adenoviruses and adeno-associated viruses being current favourites, it might be possible to aerosolize the delivery system, penetrate recipient epithelial cells and achieve a degree of appropriate protein expression. There has been similar speculation about the possibility of inserting the α_1-antitrypsin gene into T-lymphocytes and delivering them by aerosol as a treatment for emphysema that occurs frequently in α_1-antitrypsin-deficient homozygotes.

DELIVERY SYSTEMS
Over the past decade many techniques have been developed for the introduction of DNA into mammalian cells (Table 9.4). Most of the non-viral methods are extremely inefficient, the exceptions being electroporation and laser micropuncture. Here the long-term viability and possible damage to endogenous DNA has yet to be assessed. For this reason, most attention has been paid to what have been called Nature's syringes, DNA and RNA viruses, and, in particular, a range of cleverly engineered retroviruses.

Evolution has tailored retroviruses to subvert the machinery of a host cell in such a way that it makes large numbers of infectious virions, which are then exported to infect other host cells. The efficiency of integration is high in dividing cells and only single copies of the insert are incorporated. The problems for gene therapy are therefore two: to modify the retrovirus so that it carries a copy of the desired gene; and to disable it in such a way that it no longer produces infectious virions but instead expresses products of the added gene.

Ingenious constructs have now been developed to solve these particular problems. The normal retroviral genome contains sequences necessary for infection, integration and transcriptional control that are in long terminal repeats (LTRs), *gag* sequences, which encode internal structural proteins of the virion core, *pol* genes, which encode a reverse transcriptase, and *env* genes, which control envelope glycoproteins on the virion membrane (Fig. 9.10). There is, additionally, a packaging sequence, which allows viral genome to be packaged into virions. The retrovirus can be disabled by removing the packaging sequence. A second recombinant virus is then constructed, with the packaging sequence intact, but with *gag*, *pol* and *env* sequences removed and replaced by the gene to be transfected together with a dominant selectable marker such as the neomycin-resistance gene. Sequential or simultaneous infection of a host cell with the two constructs (helper and recombinant) is then carried out. The recombinant vector uses the signals from the helper for integration and replication, and its own packaging sequences to package its own RNA into recombinant virus. Although the recombinant virus can infect and integrate into the DNA of other dividing cells, it does not give rise to additional infectious virions. The selectable marker makes it possible to grow modified cells in a medium that kills off host cells that have not been transfected.

Adenoviruses and adeno-associated viruses (AAV) are also being explored as potential vectors for gene transfer. The latter have a number of advantages over retroviruses, including the fact that they are ubiquitous in humans and can be concentrated in culture to very high titres. They appear to be non-pathogenic and may actually play a role in preventing disease. AAVs are naturally defective and require co-infection with helper adenoviruses or herpes viruses for replication of their 5 kb single-stranded DNA. However, there is still a critical lack of information on their mechanism of integration into host cells and the long-term consequences of their use in mammalian systems.

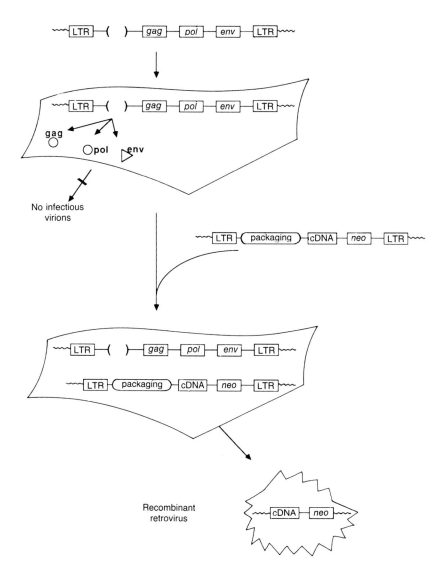

Fig. 9.10. The combined use of a disabled helper retrovirus (at top) and a recombinant retrovirus (at the right), containing cDNA from the gene of interest to transfect recipient cells. See the text for details.

APPROPRIATE EXPRESSION

Some genes are expressed at low levels in a large variety of cell types (housekeeping genes), while others have a more specialized expression both in terms of tissue and also of time during development. Unfortunately most of the more common 'solved' genetic diseases are based on specialized genes. The haemoglobinopathies are an obvious example; globin genes are expressed in only red cells and there has to be synchronous production of α- and β-globin chains to avoid a thalassaemia phenotype. Although much has been learned recently about the regulatory elements that direct high-level tissue-specific expression of globin genes, retrovirus-mediated transduction into mouse bone marrow cells seems to lead either to short-lived expression of globin or to a waxing and waning phenomenon. For the present, it would seem sensible to concentrate on the very much less common severe immunodeficiency disorders, where tissue-specific regulation is less likely to be important.

AVOIDING DAMAGE

Any clinical trials of gene therapy will eventually have to be conducted with imperfect knowledge of the potential damaging effects of introducing exogenous genes and their vectors. Random integration has the obvious capacity to interrupt the function of normal genes and to activate the expression of inappropriate genes, for example, cellular oncogenes. Recently there has been a flurry of studies on targetted gene insertion using the principle of homologous recombination between exogenous DNA and chromosomal DNA containing the defective gene (Fig. 9.11). In principle this permits the introduction of a correcting sequence into exactly the right site, and the possibility of stable and appropriate expression. In practice, the efficiency of gene targetting is still too low for it to be anything other than a remote clinical possibility.

DO WE NEED GENE THERAPY?

It is apparent that the prospect of gene therapy is not likely to be realized in the near future and that there are still large technical problems to be overcome. Where alternative treatments are available it will be difficult to justify highly experimental gene-transfer approaches unless they are likely to be significantly more successful. However, many common genetic diseases, such as the muscular dystrophies, fragile X syndrome, Huntington's disease and Tay–Sachs disease, have a truly dismal prognosis, and there seems little

266

prospect of alternative therapies being developed. Here the only current option is avoidance by prenatal diagnosis. An exchange of comments in the journal *Nature* highlights the dilemma. 'An efficient method for transfecting haematopoietic stem cells offers major encouragement to those who believe that the ultimate goal of clinical genetics is gene replacement therapy.' (Weatherall, 1984). 'People do not want their babies to be medical successes. The ultimate goal of

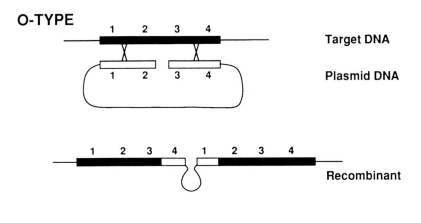

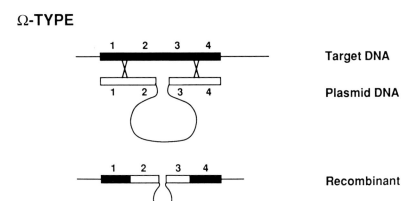

Fig. 9.11. Gene targetting by homologous recombination. The plasmid DNA contains the exogenous sequences to be inserted, whose positioning is directed by complementarity to the target DNA. In O-type recombination, sequences are added to the target DNA, whereas in Ω-type recombination, new sequences replace complementary sequences in the target DNA.

267

clinical genetics is to assist couples in having normal children.'
(Pembrey, 1985). Although these views may seem poles apart, it is
possible to reconcile them. At present, the most important approach
to genetic diseases is to try to avoid them by delivering widescale
programmes of prenatal diagnosis and screening. In the longer term,
some attempt must be made to provide effective treatment for those
who drop through the prenatal diagnosis and screening net or whose
parents found the prospect of termination of pregnancy ethically
unacceptable.

THE HUMAN GENOME PROJECT

In the mid 1980s – the precise time is difficult to pinpoint, although it
is often attributed to a meeting in Santa Cruz in 1985 – the idea
emerged of sequencing the entire human genome, all 3×10^9 base-
pairs contained within 24 different chromosomes. It was a proposal
that fuelled an immediate and continuing controversy. Some biologists could see their prospects of attracting research grants being
diminished by the siphoning-off of funds to support a mega-science
and, perhaps, centrally directed programme. Systems analysts
wondered how the gargantuan flow of information could be col-
lected, recorded and made accessible. Seasoned molecular biologists
argued that there was little point in sequencing the entire genome
when more than 95% of it has no apparent function. Ethicists were
concerned at the possible misuse and abuse of such detailed knowledge of the genetic structure of man. National and commercial
rivalries emerged; 'Who owns the human genome?' asked an editorial
in Science in July 1987 (Roberts, 1987). Walter Gilbert, a Nobel prize
laureate who also runs a commercial company, had no doubts; the
copyright on a DNA sequence belongs to the person or interest that
carries out the sequencing and would be made available to other
parties at a price. This view was vigorously disputed, and arguments
about whether sequence data per se are patentable or should be
patented, continue to rage.

It was perhaps not surprising that, for several years, the human
genome project hung fire. However, it was apparent that mapping
and sequencing activities were already proceeding at a formidable
rate in thousands of different laboratories around the world, and that
the issue was not whether the genome should be sequenced but what
strategies should be employed, what priorities should be assigned,
and how the different efforts might be advantageously coordinated.
A number of different organizations, led by the National Institutes of
Health and the Department of Energy in the U.S.A., but including

international consortia such as HUGO (Human Genome Organiza-
tion) and national groupings, are now beginning to reach some agree-
ment on how to advance the biggest project ever attempted in the
biological sciences.

A major issue has been whether the most sensible procedure is to
start with a linkage map and then to proceed to a physical map or
whether to attempt both simultaneously. A linkage map relates genes
or cloned DNA sequences to one another along the various chromosomes; this type of mapping with respect to disease genes was
outlined in Chapter 5. It depends on the analysis of co-inheritance of
genetic loci in informative families and the statistical interpretation of
whether loci cosegregate more often than would be expected by
chance. Once two loci are found to be genetically linked, their
approximate distance from each other can be calculated from the
frequency of recombination. Groups of different loci (defined by suitable DNA polymorphisms) can be studied simultaneously by multi-
point linkage analysis and a map built up in which the distance
between markers is expressed in the unit of recombination, the centimorgan (cM). As pointed out earlier, a map unit of 1 cM cor-
responds very roughly to 1 Mb of DNA. However, recombination
frequencies per megabase of DNA vary considerably both by sex and
by chromosomal region. Overall, there are higher frequencies of
recombination in female meioses than in male meioses (though not in
all chromosomal regions), so that linkage maps in females have
greater apparent distances. Telomeric regions of chromosomes
undergo proportionately more recombination events in males
whereas centromeric regions undergo more recombination events in
females. Thus the rough, 10 cM linkage map of the human genome
that already exists has uneven and uncertain spacing, and needs to be
backed up by physical characterization. The ultimate resolution of a
linkage map is of the order of 1 cM, although there will often be larger
gaps owing to the absence of suitable polymorphic markers (Fig.
9.12).

Physical maps of the genome are based on either cytogenetic or
molecular technologies. Cytogenetically based maps order loci with
respect to the visible banding patterns along chromosomes, using
data from somatic cell hybrids or the increasingly sensitive techniques
of in situ hybridization (Chapter 7). Molecular maps characterize
large tracts of DNA on the basis of landmarks established by restriction endonuclease cleavage. DNA fragments are cloned in suitable
vectors and the different clones related to one another by virtue of
overlapping restriction sites or sequences, to give a set of contiguous

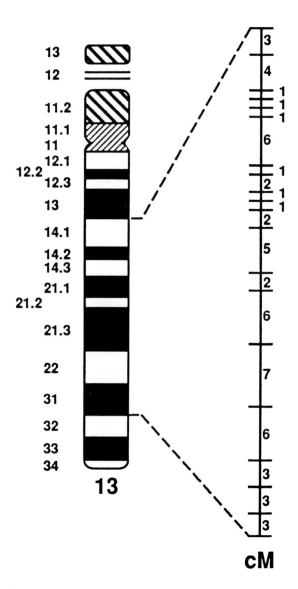

Fig. 9.12. A sex-averaged linkage map of part of chromosome 13q, showing how difficult it is to close the gaps to achieve the theoretical 1 cM limit of resolution. This represents the most comprehensive map of the region yet achieved.

DNA pieces or a contig map. The advent of vectors such as yeast artificial chromosomes (YACs), capable of handling DNA fragments up to 500 kb in size, is now permitting considerably larger contig maps to be created in specific chromosomal regions (Fig. 9.13).

Investigators creating contig maps often sequence portions of the DNA in their overlapping clones, perhaps in the search for a gene of interest or to ensure that clones are, indeed, overlapping. Thus some portions of the human genome have already been sequenced, even though these are a minute fraction of the total genomic DNA and are distributed at random amongst the chromosomes. One of the issues that has exercised proponents of the human genome project has been how to relate the different sequences to one another to build an overall map. A particular contig map depends on the physical existence of a clone collection, which may then have to be transferred to another laboratory to establish or rule out a possible relationship to another contig map. If clone collections are unavailable or if they degenerate in storage, it will be difficult to establish continuity in the creation of the physical map.

This problem has now been resolved by the ingenious idea of using a common language for landmarks in the human genome. Any sequence of 200 to 500 bp of genomic DNA that can be amplified specifically by the polymerase chain reaction (PCR) constitutes a land-mark or sequence-tagged site (STS). These sequences, together with the data on the most appropriate primers for PCR amplification, will be recorded in an STS databank (Fig. 9.14). An investigator who had constructed a contig map for a particular chromosomal region could test the map for relationships with other defined regions of the genome simply by looking for an established STS with primer data from the STS databank. If the average spacing of the STSs was 100 kb (a fragment size suitable for YAC cloning) some 30 000 sites would be necessary. It is estimated that about one-half of these already exist.

A broad strategy of the human genome project might therefore be to advance on two parallel fronts. A short-term goal would be to improve the resolution of the linkage map to a spacing of about 2 cM, with no gaps greater than 5 cM. This would provide a framework for physical mapping, the assembly of continuous regions of at least 2 Mb of DNA, each containing some 20 or more STSs as reference landmarks. The longer-term goal of systematic sequencing of whole regions or even chromosomes could be postponed until later. As methods of automatic sequencing improve, perhaps to the level of 1000 kb per day (currently it is probably less than 2 kb per day) it will become a practical prospect to sequence the entire human genome in a 10 to 15 year period.

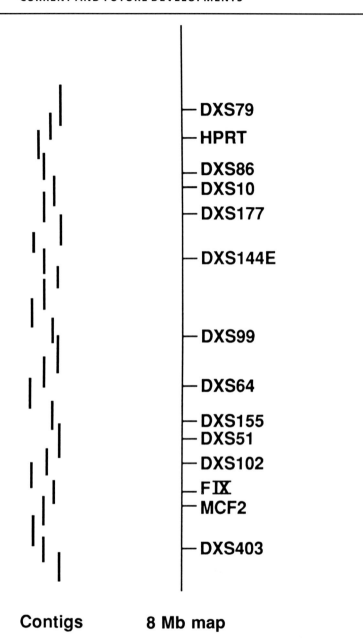

Contigs   **8 Mb map**

Fig. 9.13. An 8 Mb physical map of region Xq26 constructed from overlapping YAC clones (contigs), shown schematically at the left. The approximate distances between markers are indicated by the scale of the vertical axis at the right.

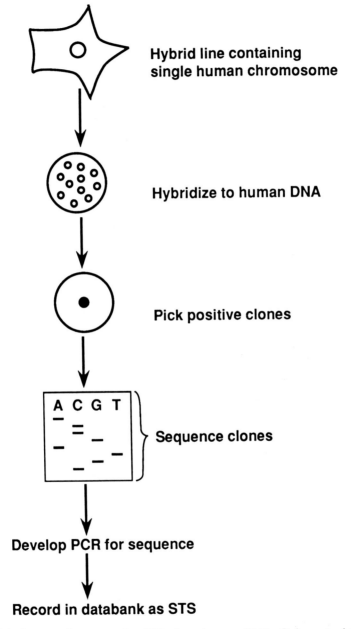

**Hybrid line containing
single human chromosome**

Hybridize to human DNA

Pick positive clones

A C G T

Sequence clones

Develop PCR for sequence

Record in databank as STS

Fig. 9.14. Strategy for generating STSs from human DNA. Only part of the clone needs to be sequenced to generate data for the PCR and to provide data for an STS bank.

273

There are, however, still alternative views as to whether this is the best strategy. Many investigators regard the long-term plan of sequencing the entire genome as something that should be postponed in favour of concentrating on transcribed genes, representing the biologically interesting 2% to 3% of the total DNA sequence. One way of doing this is to select clones from cDNA libraries, which theoretically contain the exon sequences of all the genes expressed in the tissue from which the library was constructed, and to sequence a 400 to 500 bp stretch of each clone. This gives enough information on the gene to allow a search to be made for homologies to known genes recorded in various sequence databanks. If no homologies are found, the sequence represents part of a newly discovered transcribed gene, and enough data are available from the partial sequence (referred to as an expressed sequence tag or EST) to allow other investigators to recognize the gene in their work. In many ways the strategy is similar to the STS concept but with landmarks in only transcribed genes and with no attempt to link the segments (either physically or genetically).

Critics of the EST approach point out that cDNA libraries do not necessarily contain representative clones from all transcribed genes in a particular tissue. Some genes may be transcribed at limited stages of development so that the mRNA is not captured in the library. Other genes exist in multiple copies leading to redundant sequencing of identical clones. Families of very similar genes might be difficult to distinguish with partial sequencing, and some members of the family might thus be missed completely. cDNA sequencing gives no information on the all-important promoter and control regions at the 5' end of the gene, since these are not transcribed. On the other hand, initial experiments, using a human brain cDNA library, have revealed a very high proportion of clones for which partial sequencing indicated they were transcribed from genes without homologies to sequences deposited in various databanks. These newly discovered genes, which have obvious importance in the biology of brain function, would not have been recognized as such by random total sequencing of stretches of genomic DNA. Thus some cDNA sequencing may be necessary to distinguish transcribed from non-transcribed components of the genome.

It is therefore likely that the human genome project will proceed with a number of complementary strategies. Establishment of a detailed linkage map is of immediate importance in providing a framework into which disease genes can be placed with greater certainty. cDNA sequencing with EST landmarks has the capacity to describe transcribed genes of significance in the biology of different tissues. But ultimately the goal remains the sequencing of the entire human genome, filling in the regions that are not transcribed, and ultimately answering the question as to whether the bulk of the genome is indeed without function.

IMPLICATIONS OF THE HUMAN GENOME PROJECT

In the discussions about whether and how to sequence the human genome there has inevitably been a fair amount of hyperbole. The statement by James Watson (1990) 'the genetic messages encoded within our DNA molecules will provide the ultimate answers to the chemical underpinnings of human existence' may seem far fetched, and was probably directed more at funding agencies than at his fellow biologists. None the less, it contains an important truth: knowing the sequences of all the genes that operate in a tissue will have a profound impact on the understanding of cell growth, differentiation and function and the ways in which these may go wrong. An indication of this potential can be seen in the speed with which cancer biologists have embraced molecular genetics and brought it to bear on the complexities of their specialty. It is the realization that the functioning of all organisms, from microbes to humans, is the direct consequence of the message of the genes, as well as the knowledge that we now have the power to decode the messages, that drives the human genome project forward. But we should not deceive ourselves into believing that knowing all the sequences will answer the major social questions of human existence. Jones (1991) makes the point in a sarcastic comment 'Once we have sequenced ourselves, we will know, apparently, which wine to buy, whether to learn a musical instrument and even whom to sleep with. The gene sequencers are pursuing the ultimate reductionist programme: to understand the message we just have to put all the letters in order.' He goes on to suggest that all the pieces of information, when put together, may make no sense at all.

This is unduly pessimistic; there is no doubt that the individual messages of the genes make a great deal of sense and are already being pressed into clinical service in prenatal diagnosis, carrier detection and genetic screening. I have more sympathy with the point of view held by those that worry not so much about meaningless messages but rather about misunderstood or misconstrued messages, in other words, the potential for abusing and misusing genetic information. The key question here is who has the right to know the genetic constitution of a particular individual?

This is not an easy question to answer and will become more

275

difficult as the flood of genetic information increases. The instinctive and reflex response is to feel that everyone has an absolute moral right to protect their own genetic privacy, in the same way as their right to protect their social privacy. And yet we have already allowed that right of genetic privacy to be qualified in important ways. Most of us do not object to insurance firms and even employers asking whether our parents are still alive, and if not, when they died and of what. If my father had died at age 42 of coronary heart disease, an insurance company might feel justified in modifying my life insurance premiums; if he had died of Huntington's disease they might well deny me a policy altogether. An insurance company would justify its actions on the grounds that I am a bad risk and that accepting bad risks throws an additional financial burden on other better-risk contributors. In actual fact, since all insurance is a form of gambling the company is merely trying not to disadvantage itself with respect to its competitors. This issue could be fairly simply resolved, if we had the will, by a tightly worded genetic discrimination Act that outlawed any genetic-type questions in an insurer's or employer's questionnaire.

It is very much more difficult to answer the question about genetic privacy when concealment clearly endangers other people. The prototype situation for this type of concern is presymptomatic testing for Huntington's disease. A person with an affected parent who wishes to know whether he or she is a gene carrier, so that responsible decisions about reproduction can be made, often needs genotype information from more distant members of the family. If such information is refused, geneticists usually accept the principle of genetic privacy and make no attempt to compel its release, even though they know that concealment can have drastic effects on future generations. Perhaps we are too sensitive to individual rights in such clearcut situations. But undoubtedly we are influenced by 'thin end of the wedge' or 'camel's nose' arguments, and fear that legal compulsion might be a precedent for much less predictable scenarios. Should a cancer patient with a p53 germ-line mutation be compelled to inform all members of the immediate family that they, too, may have a high risk of cancer? What about a woman who is carrying a fragile X premutation? These are just a few of the proliferating collection of susceptibility genes, whose existence in families and populations raises the most difficult problems about the limits to genetic privacy.

In the face of these types of issue, one might ask whether we are ready for a Human Genome Project. The answer is that we are probably not and that ethical analysis and public scrutiny have already fallen well behind the technical advances. Although this is regrettable, it is not likely to be fatal. Human genome mapping is now such an integral part of molecular genetic research that it is inconceivable that it could be stopped in its tracks. Either it will occur as a series of individual initiatives in the thousands of high-technology laboratories around the world or it will be a coordinated and integrated approach. The growing signs that it will be the latter bring it into the realm of public science and ensure that the prospects and achievements are fully reported and answerable to the public good.

SUGGESTED READING
AVOIDANCE OF GENETIC DISEASE

Brock, D. J. H. (1978). Screening for neural tube defects. In: Scrimgeour, J. B. (Editor), *Towards the Prevention of Fetal Malformation*, pp. 37–48, Edinburgh University Press, Edinburgh.

Brock, D. J. H. (1982). *Early Diagnosis of Fetal Defects*. Churchill Livingstone, Edinburgh.

Brock, D. J. H., Curtis, A., Barron, L., Dinwoodie, D., Crosbie, A., Mennie, M., *et al.* (1989). Predictive testing for Huntington's disease with linked DNA markers. *Lancet* **ii:** 463–466.

Brock, D. J. H., Shrimpton, A. E., Jones, C. and McIntosh, I. (1991). Cystic fibrosis: the new genetics, *Journal of the Royal Society of Medicine* **84:** 2–6.

Edwards, J. H., Lyon, M. F. and Southern, E. M. (Editors), (1988). *The Prevention and Avoidance of Genetic Disease*. The Royal Society, London.

Emery, A. E. H. and Miller, J. R. (Editors), (1976). *Registers for the Detection and Prevention of Genetic Disease*. Stratton, New York.

Ferguson-Smith, M. A. and Yates, J. R. W. (1984). Maternal age-specific rates for chromosome aberrations and factors influencing them. *Prenatal Diagnosis* **4:** 5–44.

Harper, P. S. (1986). The prevention of Huntington's chorea. *Journal of the Royal College of Physicians of London* **20:** 7–14.

Milunsky, A. (Editor), (1986). *Genetic Disorders and the Fetus: Diagnosis, Prevention and Treatment*. 2nd Edition, Plenum Press, New York.

Monk, M. (1992). Preimplantation diagnosis – a comprehensive review. In: Brock, D. J. H., Rodeck, C. H. and Ferguson-Smith, M. A. (Editors), *Prenatal Diagnosis and Screening*, pp. 627–637, Churchill Livingston, London.

Rodeck, C. H. (Editor), (1987). *Fetal Diagnosis of Genetic Defects*. Bailliere Tindall, London.

Skraastad, M. I., Verwest, A., Bakker, E., Vegter-van der Vlis, M., van Leeuwen-Cornelisse, I., Roos, R. A. C., *et al.* (1991). Presymptomatic, prenatal, and exclusion testing for Huntington's disease using 7 closely linked DNA markers. *American Journal of Medical Genetics* **38**: 217–222.

Vogel, F. and Motulsky, A. G. (1986). *Human Genetics: Problems and Approaches*. Springer-Verlag, Berlin.

Wald, N. J. (Editor), (1984). *Antenatal and Neonatal Screening*. Oxford University Press, Oxford.

Wald, N. J. (1991). Couple screening for cystic fibrosis. *Lancet* **338**: 1318–1320.

GENE THERAPY

Beaudet, A. L., Mulligan, R. and Verma, I. M. (Editors), (1989). *Gene Transfer and Gene Therapy*. Alan R. Liss, New York.

Capecchi, M. R. (1989). Altering the genome by homologous recombination. *Science* **244**: 1288–1292.

Culliton, B. J. (1989). A genetic shield to prevent emphysema. *Science* **246**: 750–751.

Davis, B. D. (1990). Limits to genetic intervention in humans: somatic and germ line. In: *Human Genetic Information: Science, Law and Ethics*. Ciba Foundation Symposium 149, pp. 91–92, John Wiley, Chichester.

Ferry, N., Duplessis, O., Houssin, D., Danos, O. and Heard, J.-M. (1991). Retroviral-mediated gene transfer into hepatocytes *in vivo*. *Proceedings of the National Academy of Sciences, U.S.A.* **88**: 8377–8381.

Friedmann, T. (1989). Progress towards human gene therapy. *Science* **244**: 1275–1281.

Kantoff, P. W., Freeman, S. M. and Anderson, F. W. (1988). Prospects for gene therapy for immunodeficiency diseases. *Annual Review of Immunology* **6**: 581–594.

Pembrey, M. E. (1985). Do we need gene therapy? *Nature (London)* **311**: 200.

Smithies, O., Gregg, R. G., Boggs, S. S., Koralewski, M. A. and Kucherlapati, R. S. (1985). Insertion of DNA sequences into the human chromosomal β globin locus by homologous recombination. *Nature (London)* **317**: 230–234.

St Louis, D. and Verma, I. M. (1988). An alternative approach to somatic cell gene therapy. *Proceedings of the National Academy of Sciences, U.S.A.* **85**: 3150–3154.

Varmus, H. (1988). Retroviruses. *Science* **240**: 1427–1435.

Vega, M. A. (1991). Prospects for homologous recombination in human gene therapy. *Human Genetics* **87:** 245–253.

Verma, I. M. (1990). Gene therapy. *Scientific American (November)* 34–41.

Williams, D. A. and Orkin, S. H. (1986). Somatic gene therapy: current status and future prospects. *Journal of Clinical Investigation* **77:** 1053–1056.

Weatherall, D. J. (1984). A step nearer gene therapy? *Nature (London)* **310:** 451.

Weatherall, D. J. (1991). Gene therapy in perspective. *Nature (London)* **349:** 275–276.

THE HUMAN GENOME PROJECT

Adams, M. D., Kelley, J. M., Gocayne, J. D., Dubnick, M., Polymeropoulos, M. H., Xiao, H., *et al.* (1991). Complementary DNA sequencing: expressed sequenced tags and human genome project. *Science* **252:** 1651–1656.

Cantor, C. R. (1990). Orchestrating the human genome project. *Science* **248:** 49–51.

Davis, B. D., Amos, H., Beckwith, J., Collier, R. J., Desrosiers, R. C., Fields, B. N., *et al.* (1990). The human genome and other initiatives. *Science* **249:** 342–343.

Dulbecco, R. (1986). A turning point in cancer research: sequencing the human genome. *Science* **231:** 1055–1056.

Editorial (1991). Free trade in human sequence data? *Nature (London)* **354:** 171–172.

Friedmann, T. (1990). The human genome project – some implications of extensive reverse genetic medicine. *American Journal of Human Genetics* **46:** 407–414.

Hunkapiller, T., Kaiser, R. J., Koop, B. F. and Hood, L. (1991). Large-scale and automated DNA sequence determination. *Science* **254:** 59–67.

Jones, J. S. (1991). Songs in the key of life. *Nature (London)* **354:** 323.

Maddox, J. (1991). The case for the human genome. *Nature (London)* **352:** 11–14.

Olson, M., Hood, L., Cantor, C. and Botstein, D. (1989). A common language for physical mapping of the human genome. *Science* **245:** 1434–1435.

Roberts, L. (1987). Who owns the human genome? *Science* **237:** 358–361.

Siniscalo, M. (1987). On the strategies and priorities for sequencing the human genome: a personal view. *Trends in Genetics* **3:** 182–184.

Stephens, J. C., Cavanaugh, M. L., Gradie, M. I., Mador, M. L. and Kidd, K. K. (1990). Mapping the human genome: current status. *Science* **250**: 237–250.

Watson, J. D. (1990). The human genome project: past, present and future. *Science* **248**: 44–49.

Wills, C. (1991). *Exons, Introns and Talking Genes: the Science Behind the Human Genome Project*. Basic Books, New York.

INDEX

transcription of DNA into RNA, 29–
  33
  ectopic, 109–12
transcriptional mutations, 93
transfection experiments, 149–50
transitions, 85
translation of RNA into protein,
  33–5
translocations, X–autosome, 178
transversion, 85
trinucleotide repeats,
  fragile X, 202–3
  Kennedy disease, 233–4
triploidy, 18–19, 181, 182
trisomy, 21, 22, 196–200
  see also Down syndrome
  maternal age and, 196
tumours
  clonality, 140–1
  suppressor genes, 149–64
    oncogenes and, 162–4
    p53, 156–61
Turner syndrome, 19, 191
twin concordance rates, 22–3

uniparental disomy, 181–2, 183–5
uracil, 29
unveitis, acute anterior, 211

variable number of tandem repeat
  polymorphisms (VNTR), 96, 97,
  99

von Hippel–Lindau syndrome, 138,
  158
von Recklinghausen disease see
  neurofibromatosis
von Willebrand disease, prenatal
  diagnosis, 249

Waardenberg syndrome, 237
WAGR syndrome, 154, 158, 205
Watson–Crick base-pairing, 26, 195
Wilms' tumour, 138, 154–5, 158,
  170(colour Fig.), 186

X chromosomes, 7
  inactivation (lyonization), 13–15,
    176–9
    model, 180
  autosome translocations, 178
X-linked ichthyosis, 134, 176
X-linked inheritance, 13–15
X-linked recessives, current status,
  134
xeroderma pigmentosum, 138, 139
Xg blood group, 176
XIST gene, 179

Y chromosomes, 7
YAC libraries, 67–9
yeast artificial chromosomes (YAC),
  67, 202

ZFY, 191